THE TAO OF
NATURAL BREATHING

For Health, Well-Being
and Inner Growth

Dennis Lewis

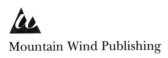

Mountain Wind Publishing

The translation from Lao Tsu on page 9 is reprinted from *Tao Te Ching* by Lao Tsu, trans., Feng/English, Copyright (c) 1972 by Gia-fu Feng and Jane English. Reprinted by permission of Alfred A Knopf Inc.

The translations from Lao Tzu on pages 21 and 113 are reprinted from *The Complete Works of Lao Tzu* by Ni, Hua Ching. Reprinted by permission of Seven Star Communications, 1996.

The translation from Lao Tzu on page 84 is reprinted from *Tao Te Ching* by Lao Tzu, trans., Victor H. Mair. Reprinted by permission of Bantam Books.

The passage by Tzu Kuo Shih on page 85 is reprinted from *Qi Gong Therapy: The Chinese Art of Healing with Energy* by Tzu Kuo Shih. Reprinted by permission of Station Hill Press.

The translations from Chuang Tzu on pages 99 and 113-14 are reprinted from *Basic Writings of Chuang Tzu* edited by Burton Watson, copyright 1964 by Columbia University Press. Reprinted by permission of the publisher.

Mountain Wind Publishing
P. O. Box 31376
San Francisco, CA 94131

Book Design: Ingalls & Associates
Designers: Caroline Byrne and Thomas Ingalls
Illustrations: Juan Li

Publisher's Cataloging in Publication
Lewis, Dennis.
The Tao of natural breathing : for health, well-being and inner growth / Dennis Lewis. — 1st ed.
p. cm.
Includes bibliographical references and index.
LCCN: 96-75684
ISBN 0-9651611-0-2

1. Breathing exercises. 2. Taoism.   I. Title.

RA782.L49 1996   613'.192
                                                       QBI96-20294
Printed in the United States of America.
3rd printing 2000.

A WORD OF CAUTION
The practices in this book are not intended to replace the services of your physician, or to provide an alternative to professional medical treatment. This book offers no diagnosis of or treatment for any specific medical problem that you may have. Where it suggests the possible usefulness of certain practices in relation to certain illnesses or symptoms, it does so solely for educational purposes—either to explore the possible relationship of natural breathing to health, or to expose the reader to alternative healing approaches from other traditions, especially the Taoist tradition of China. The breathing practices outlined in this book are extremely gentle, and should—if carried out as described—be beneficial to your overall physical and psychological health. If you have any serious medical or psychological problem, however—such as heart disease, high blood pressure, cancer, mental illness, or recent abdominal or chest surgery—you should consult your physician before undertaking any of these practices.

Dedicated to my son, Benoit, who, from the moment of his birth, has inspired me to always attempt to keep learning and growing.

And with my most profound gratitude to Lord John Pentland, my primary teacher, who was an outstanding leader of the Gurdjieff Work in America until his death in 1984, and who taught me how to think from the perspective and sensation of wholeness; Jean Klein, the Advaita Vedanta master who helped me understand that love and consciousness are at the very heart of being; and Mantak Chia, the Taoist master who brought the Healing Tao to America, and who, along with Chi Nei Tsang practitioner Gilles Marin, showed me that healing is a power we all have—the creative power of life itself.

CONTENTS

Empty yourself of everything.

Let the mind become still.

The ten thousand things rise and fall while the Self watches
   their return.

They grow and flourish and then return to the source.

Returning to the source is stillness, which is the way of nature....

Lao Tsu, *Tao Te Ching*

FOREWORD

There is a growing interest today in the relationship of breathing to health and spiritual development. Unfortunately, few people who experiment with their breath understand the importance of "natural breathing." This is the kind of spontaneous, whole-body breathing that one can observe in an infant or a young child. Instead of trying to learn to breathe naturally, many people impose complicated breathing techniques on top of their already bad breathing habits. These habits are not in harmony with the psychological and physiological laws of the mind and body. They are not in harmony with the Tao.

Natural breathing is an integral part of the Tao. For thousands of years Taoist masters have taught natural breathing to their students through chi kung, tai chi, and various other meditative and healing arts and sciences. Through natural breathing we are able to support our overall health. We are able to improve the functioning and efficiency of our heart, lungs, and other internal organs and systems. We are able to help balance our emotions. We are able to transform our stress and negativity into the energy that we can use for self-healing and self-development. And we are better able to extract and absorb the energy we need for spiritual growth and independence.

Many books on breathing have been published over the past several years. None of them, however, has gone as deeply into the meaning, practice, and benefits of natural breathing as this important new work by Dennis Lewis. Based on his own long study and research in various traditions and disciplines, including the Healing Tao, Lewis brings together in one book the psychosomatic vision, the scientific knowledge, and the vital practices that can help us discover the power of natural breathing to rejuvenate and transform our lives.

The Tao of Natural Breathing makes a big contribution to our understanding of how the way we breathe influences our lives. Whatever their level of experience, readers will gain new insights into their own specific breathing habits and how these habits often undermine their health and well-being. They will understand that natural, authentic breathing depends less on learning new breathing techniques than it does on what Lewis calls the "reeducation" of our inner perception. This reeducation, which involves learning how to sense the inner structures and energies of the mind and body, lies at the heart of the Taoist approach to healing and spiritual development.

MASTER MANTAK CHIA
The International Healing Tao
Chiang Mai, Thailand

PREFACE

William Blake wrote: "There is a crack in everything that God has made." For me, this crack—this place where something new and more meaningful can enter our lives—became especially visible in 1990, when I found myself physically, emotionally, and spiritually exhausted, with a constant, sharp pain on the right side of my rib cage. I had just gone through the enormous stress of selling my public relations agency to a well-known English firm, and had worked to maximize the sale price of the company for two years under the direction of the new owners. Though I had had chronic abdominal discomfort for many years, and indeed had been diagnosed with "colitis" some years before, this pain was different. I went to doctors, massage therapists, and various body-work practitioners to put an end to it, but to no avail. It was during this period that I met Gilles Marin, a student of Taoist master Mantak Chia, and a teacher and practitioner of Chi Nei Tsang (CNT), a Taoist healing practice using internal-organ chi massage and work with breathing to clear unhealthy tensions and energies from our bodies.

When Gilles first put his hands into my belly and began to massage my inner organs and tissues, and when he began to ask me to breathe into parts of myself that I had never experienced through my breath, I had no idea of the incredible journey of discovery that I was beginning. Though Gilles told me that CNT was part of a larger system of healing and spiritual practices called the "Healing Tao," founded by Master Chia, my immediate concern was simply to get rid of the pain. I had my own spiritual practices; what I needed was healing.

Healing. ... A word I had not pondered very deeply in my life. But as Gilles began to work more intensively with me, and as it became increasingly clear that the healing process depended in large part on my own inner awareness, I began to understand why the expressions "to heal" and "to make whole" have the same roots. Though the physical pain disappeared after several sessions, and though I began to feel more alive, a deeper, psychic pain began to emerge—the pain of recognizing that in spite of all my efforts over many years toward self-knowledge and self-transformation, I had managed to open myself to only a small portion of the vast scale of the physical, emotional, and spiritual energies available to us at every moment. As Gilles continued working on me, and as my breath began to penetrate deeper into myself, I began to sense layer after layer of tension, anger, fear, and sadness resonating in my abdomen below the level of my so-called waking consciousness, and consuming the energies I needed not only for health, but also for a real engagement with life. And this deepening sensation at the very center of my being, painful as it was, brought with it an opening not only in the tissues of my belly, but also in my most intimate attitudes toward myself, a welcoming of hitherto unconscious fragments of myself into a new sense of discovery, wholeness, and inner growth.

I quickly realized that Chi Nei Tsang—with its penetration into my physical and emotional energies through touch and breathwork—provided a direct, healing pathway into myself, and as I learned more about it through its action on me I soon found myself taking classes from Gilles and even beginning to work on my friends. I also found myself taking classes in healing practices and chi kung, many of which involved special breathing practices, from various Healing Tao teachers, including Master Chia. After more than a year of CNT classes and many hours of clinical practice, I was tested by Master Chia and certified by him to do CNT professionally. And after many Healing Tao classes and retreats, as well as intensive work on myself, I also became certified by Master Chia to teach some of the Healing Tao practices. Since then I have done CNT work both on my own clients and at a Chinese medicine clinic in San Francisco, and have taught ongoing Healing Tao classes and workshops, with a large emphasis on breathing.

As a result of my work with the Healing Tao, as well as with other teachings, such as the Gurdjieff Work and Advaita Vedanta, two facts have become clear to me with regard to the relationship of breath to health and inner growth. First, that our poor breathing habits have arisen not only out of our psychosomatic "ig-norance," our lack of organic awareness, but also out of our unconscious need for a buffering mechanism to keep us from sensing and feeling the reality of our own deep-rooted fears and contradictions. There is absolutely no doubt that *superficial breathing ensures a superficial experience of ourselves.* Second, that if we were able to breathe "naturally" for even a small percentage of the more than 15,000 breaths we take during each waking day we would be taking a huge step not only toward preventing many of the physical and psychological problems that have become endemic to modern life, but also toward supporting our own inner growth—the growth of awareness of who and what we really are, of our own essential being. It is my hope that the ideas and practices explored in this book will help make this possible.

Introduction

A Miracle and a Warning

The process of breathing, of the fundamental movement of inspiration and expiration, is one of the great miracles of existence. It not only unleashes the energies of life, but it also provides a healing pathway into the deepest recesses of our being. To inhale fully is to fill ourselves with the energies of life, to be inspired; to exhale fully is to empty ourselves, to open ourselves to the unknown, to be expired. It is through a deepening awareness of the ever-changing rhythms of this primal process that we begin to awaken our inner healing powers—the energy of wholeness.

To breathe is to live. To breathe fully is to live fully, to manifest the full range and power of our inborn potential for vitality in everything that we sense, feel, think, and do. Unfortunately, few of us breathe fully. We have lost the capability of "natural breathing," a capability that we had as babies and young children. Our chronic shallow breathing reduces the working capacity of our respiratory system to only about one-third of its potential, diminishes the exchange of gases and thus the production of energy in our cells, deprives us of the many healthful actions that breathing naturally would have on our inner organs, cuts us off from our own real feelings, and promotes disharmony and "dis-ease" at every level of our lives.

What is natural breathing? How would this kind of breathing alter our lives and our health? To answer these questions we must undertake an experimental study of breathing in the laboratory of our own body. We must personally experience how our breath is intimately bound up

17

not just with our energy, but with every aspect of our being—from the health of our tissues, organs, bones, muscles, hormones, and blood to the quality and breadth of our thoughts, attitudes, emotions, and consciousness. We must begin to understand the great power that our breathing has to help open us or close us not only to our own inner healing powers but also to our potential for psychological and spiritual development.

Of all the great ancient and modern teachings that have explored the full significance of breath in our lives, the Taoist tradition of China, which is more a way of life than a formal religion, offers one of the most practical and insightful approaches to the use of breath for health and well-being. One of the reasons for this is that from the very beginning of Taoism, at the time of the reign of the Yellow Emperor (Huang Ti) around 2700 B.C., the goals of health and longevity were never separated from the goals of spiritual evolution and immortality. Taoists realized that a long, healthy life filled with vitality is not only an intelligent goal in its own right but also an important support for the more difficult goal of spiritual growth and independence. Supported by more than 4,000 years of experimentation with their own physical, emotional, mental, and spiritual energies through special postures and movements, massage, visualization, sound, meditation, diet, and many other practical disciplines, the Taoists observed that natural breathing—breathing according to the actual "laws" of the human organism—could have a powerful influence on the quantity and quality of these energies and thus on the quality and direction of our lives. For if the Tao can be defined at all, it means *the way*, the laws, of nature and the universe—the laws of creation and evolution. It is through living in harmony with these laws that we become free to discover and fulfill our physical, psychological, and spiritual destiny.

The Tao of Natural Breathing integrates key Taoist teachings and practices regarding breath—especially those arising through my work with Taoist master Mantak Chia—with my observations and discoveries over the past 30 years in relation to various other systems and teachings, including the Gurdjieff Work, Advaita Vedanta, Feldenkrais®, and Ilse Middendorf, as well as with important principles from anatomy, physiology, and neurochemistry. It is my experience that any serious work with breathing requires far more than appropriate exercises. It also requires a clear "scientific view" of the human body and a deep work of organic awareness—the ability to sense and feel oneself from the inside.

A WARNING ABOUT BREATHING EXERCISES

The great spiritual pathfinder G. I. Gurdjieff once said that "without mastering breathing nothing can be mastered."[1] But he also warned that without complete knowledge of our organism, especially of the interrelationships of the rhythms of our various organs, efforts to change our breathing can bring great harm. It is clear that work with breathing, especially some of the advanced yogic breathing techniques (pranayama) taught in the West through both classes and books, is fraught with many dangers. In his book *Hara: The Vital Center of Man*, Karlfried Durckheim—a pioneer in the integration of body, mind, and spirit—discusses some of the dangers of teaching yogic breathing techniques to Westerners. He points out that most of these exercises, which "imply tension," were designed for Indians, who suffer from "an inert letting-go." Westerners, on the other hand, suffer from "too much upward pull ... too much will." Durckheim states that even though many yoga teachers try to help their students relax before giving them breathing exercises, they do not realize that the "letting-go" required for deep relaxation can be achieved "only after long practice." At best, says Durckheim, giving breathing exercises prematurely grafts new tensions onto the already established ones, and brings about "an artificially induced vitality ... followed by a condition of exhaustion and the aspirant discontinues his efforts, his practice."[2]

Based on my own work on myself, as well as on my observation of others, I believe that it is only after many months (or even years) of progressive practice rooted in self-observation and self-awareness that most Westerners can experience the deep inner relaxation, the freedom from willfulness, needed to benefit in a lasting way from advanced breathing exercises—whether yogic, Taoist, or otherwise. Breathing exercises involving complicated counting schemes, alternate nostril breathing, reverse breathing, breath retention, hyperventilation,[3] and so on make sense only for people who already breathe *naturally*, making use of their entire body in the breathing process. It is my experience that natural breathing *is in itself* a powerful form of self-healing. That is why *The Tao of Natural Breathing* explores this kind of breathing in so much depth, describing in detail some fundamental perspectives and practices that can, through increased inner awareness, help us see and transform our own personal obstacles to its manifestation in our lives.

One could say, of course, as some Taoist masters and other teachers have said, that since natural breathing is natural, *any effort* to breathe naturally both misses the point and is counterproductive. They maintain that when our mind becomes calm and empty, natural breathing will arise automatically.[4] Accepting this assertion, however, does not solve the problem; it simply puts us in front of another question: what are the conditions that allow us to calm and empty our minds? What personal work is needed? It is no use to shift the problem from the body to the mind or from the mind to the body. Natural breathing involves the participation of both.

The appearance of natural breathing in our lives is not just a matter of what we do, but also—and perhaps more importantly—of how we do it. If we approach the practices in this book as mere techniques to be manipulated by our so-called will, they will bring us nothing. If, however, we can approach them as natural vehicles to explore the physiological and psychological laws of our mind and body—through direct impressions coming from an inner clarity of awareness—we may in fact begin to learn what it means to calm and empty our minds. No matter how we live or what we do (or don't do), we are always doing something; we are always practicing something—if only mechanically repeating and further entrenching the narrow, often unhealthy, habits of mind, body, and perception that shape our lives. To gain real benefit from the practices in this book, then, we must approach them as consciously as possible, taking care to *understand* their aim, *feel* their spirit, and *sense* their effect on our entire being.

EXPANDING OUR NARROW SENSE OF SELF

The real power of the ideas and practices described in this book is to help us first experience and then free ourselves from the many narrow, unconscious attitudes we have about ourselves and the world—attitudes that create stress and other problems for us in almost every area of our lives. It is often these very attitudes—deeply entrenched in our minds, hearts, and bodies, and manifested through and supported by our breathing—that diminish our awareness, constrict our life force, and prevent us from living conscious, healthy lives in harmony with ourselves, with others, and with our environment.

Fortunately, we do not have to try to deal with each of these attitudes individually—an impossible task in one lifetime. Like spokes radiating out from the central axle of a wheel, our attitudes radiate out from the axle of our own particular self-image: the narrow, incomplete, yet strong image of self, of "I," that permeates almost everything that we think, feel, and do. According to Lao Tzu, if we can somehow expand this narrow image we have of ourselves and live from our wholeness, then many of our problems will disappear on their own:

> What is meant by saying that the greatest trouble
> is the strong sense of individual self
> that people carry in all circumstances?
> People are beset with great trouble
> because they define their lives so narrowly.
> If they forsake their narrow sense of self
> and live wholly, then what can they call trouble?[5]

To see and free ourselves from our own "narrow sense of self" is to begin to become open to the tremendous healing forces and energies that create and maintain our lives—to experience for ourselves how the alchemical substances of matter and the magical ideas of mind are linked in the unified, transformative dance of yin and yang—the dynamic polarity of opposites from which all life springs. It is also to experience here and now the return to the primal, expansive emptiness and silence of "wu chi," the all-inclusive wholeness that is the source of both our being and our well-being. It is our breath that can help guide us on this remarkable journey into ourselves.

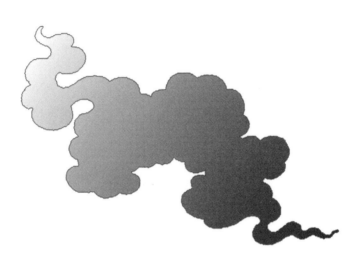

1
THE MECHANICS OF BREATHING

The process of breathing,
if we can begin to understand it
in relation to the whole of life,
shows us the way to let go
of the old and open to the new.

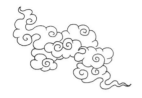

The process of breathing is a living metaphor for understanding how to expand our narrow sense of ourselves and be present to the healing energies that are both in and around us. Every time we inhale we take in some 10^{22} atoms, including approximately one million of the same atoms of air inhaled by Lao Tzu, Buddha, Christ, and everyone else who has ever lived on this earth. Every time we exhale, we return these atoms to the atmosphere to be renewed for both present and future generations. Every time we inhale, we absorb oxygen expelled into the atmosphere as a "waste product" by the earth's plant life. Every time we exhale, we expel carbon dioxide as a "waste product" into the atmosphere where it can eventually be absorbed by this same plant life. In nature, nothing is wasted. Our breath is a link in the cosmic ecology—in the conservation, transformation, and exchange of substances in nature's complex metabolism. It connects our so-called inner world with the vast scale of the outer world—of the earth and its atmosphere, as well as of all organic life—through the perceptible alternation of yin and yang, of negative and positive, of emptying and filling. The process of breathing, if we can begin to understand it in relation to the whole of life, shows us the way to let go of the old and open to the new. It shows us the way to experience who and what we actually are. It shows us the way to wholeness and well-being.

SOME PERSONAL HISTORY

In my own case, breathing took on a special, historical significance for me long before I understood why. As a child I had a tremendous fascination with holding my breath. Lying in bed, I would often hold my breath for two minutes or so before finding myself gasping for air. As a young adult, the moment I started wearing suits I realized that I was troubled by the sensation of a tight collar or a tie around my neck. It was only later, when I was in my early thirties, that my mother told me I had been a breech baby, and that the doctors had fully expected me to come into the world dead, strangled by the umbilical cord wrapped tightly around my neck. Indeed, it was wrapped around my neck, but I was still able to breathe, still able to take in the precious nectar that we call air.

It is obvious to me today, however, that my 30-hour struggle to reach light and take my first breath left deep impressions in my body and nervous system, and laid the foundation for some of the fundamental fears and insecurities that have often motivated my behavior as an adult. It is obvious to me today also that this deeply entrenched belief that only through persistence and struggle could I somehow find meaning and happiness in my life—a mode of behavior which served me well during birth, as well as during my childhood and teenage years—became an obstacle to my health and psychological growth as I grew older. All of this has become clearer as my breathing has begun to give up its restrictive hold on my sensory and emotional awareness, expanding into more of the whole of myself.

THE NEED FOR CLARITY AND MINDFULNESS

What is the relationship of our breath to our experience of ourselves and to real health and well-being? What is the relationship of our breath to our quest for self-knowledge and inner growth? To begin to answer these questions in a way that can have a long-lasting, beneficial impact on our lives, it is not enough to go to a weekend rebirthing or breathing intensive, or to simply start doing exercises from a magazine or book. Because of the intimate relationship between mind and body— the many subtle yet powerful ways they influence each other—any lasting, effective work with our breath requires *clear mental knowledge* of the mechanics of natural breathing and its relationship to our muscles, our emotions, and our thoughts. The clarity of this picture in our mind will help us become more conscious of our own individual patterns of breathing. It is through being "mindful" of these patterns that we will begin to sense and feel the various psychophysical forces acting on our breath from both the past and the present. And it is through the actual observation of these forces in our own bodies that we will begin to see how we use our breathing to buffer ourselves from physical and psychological experiences and memories too difficult or painful to confront. And, finally, it is through this entire process—the integration of mental clarity with sensory and emotional awareness—that we will begin to experience the extraordinary power of "natural breathing" and its ability to support the process of healing and wholeness in our lives.

THE ANATOMY OF BREATHING

For most of us, our cycle of inhalation and exhalation occurs at an average resting rate of 12 to 14 times a minute when we are awake, and six to eight times a minute when we are asleep. A baby breathes at about twice these rates. Our breathing rates can change dramatically in relation to what we are doing or experiencing. Under extreme physical activity or stress, for example, the rate can go up to 100 times a minute. For those who have worked seriously with their breath, the resting rate can go down to four to eight times a minute, since they take in more oxygen and expel more carbon dioxide with each inhalation and exhalation.

The Chest Cavity and Lungs

The process of breathing takes place mainly in the chest cavity, the top and sides of which are bounded by the ribs (which slant downward and forward) and the attached intercostal muscles, and the bottom by the dome-shaped muscular partition of the diaphragm (Figure 1). Inside this cavity lie the heart and the two lungs. Shaped somewhat like pyramids, the lungs are divided into three lobes on the right and two on the left. The lobes are composed of a spongy labyrinth of sacs, which, if flattened out, would cover an area of approximately 100 square yards. The lungs are covered by the pleura, a double-layer membrane lining the inside of the ribs, and are supported by the diaphragm. Extremely elastic, the lungs are free to move in any direction except where they are

Chest Cavity

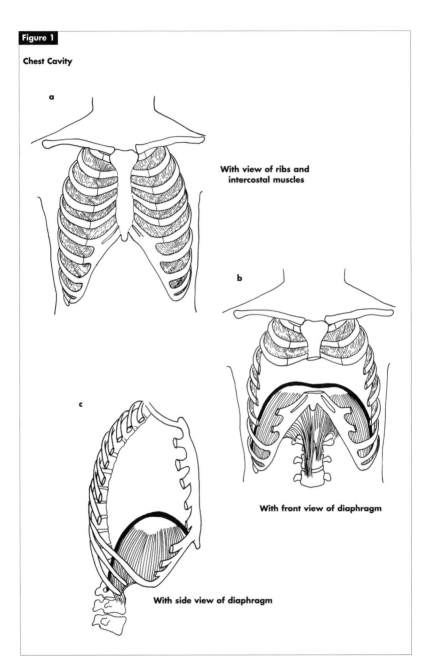

a

With view of ribs and
intercostal muscles

b

With front view of diaphragm

c

With side view of diaphragm

attached through tubes and arteries to the trachea and heart. Though the lungs have a total air capacity of about 5,000 milliliters, the average breath is only about 500 milliliters. Though, as we shall see, we can learn to exhale much more air than we normally do, no matter how fully we may exhale, the lungs always hold a reserve of about 1,000 milliliters of air to keep them from becoming completely deflated. It is easy to see that most of us use a small percentage of our lungs' capacity.

We seldom pay attention to the breathing process in the course of our daily activities, but when we do we can sense the chest cavity expanding and contracting, somewhat like a bellows. During inhalation, the rib muscles (intercostals) expand and elevate the ribs, the sternum moves slightly upward, and the diaphragm flattens downward. The expanded space creates a partial vacuum that sucks the lungs outward toward the walls of the chest and downward toward the diaphragm, thus increasing their volume as air is drawn in automatically from the outside (Figure 2). The air that we inhale is composed of about 20 percent oxygen and .03 percent carbon dioxide; the rest is nitrogen. During exhalation, the rib muscles relax, the sternum moves downward, the diaphragm relaxes upward (regaining its full dome-like curvature), and the old air is expelled upward through the trachea as the lungs recede from the walls of the chest and shrink back to their original size (Figure 3). The exhaled air consists of 16 percent oxygen and 4 percent carbon dioxide. It is saturated with water vapor produced by metabolic activity.

The Movement of Air through the Respiratory System

As air enters our nose, particles of dust and dirt are filtered out by the hairs that line our nostrils. As the air continues on through the nasal passages it is warmed and humidified by the mucous membranes of the septum, which divides the nose into two cavities. If too many particles accumulate on the membranes of the nose, we automatically secrete mucus to trap them or sneeze to expel them. In general, air does not move through the nasal passages equally at the same time. Usually when the left nostril is more open, the right one is more congested and

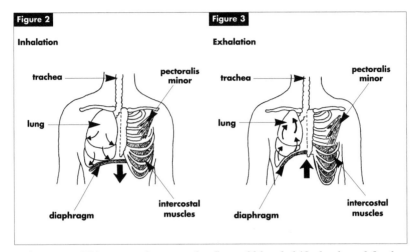

Figure 2

Inhalation

trachea

pectoralis
minor

lung

diaphragm

intercostal
muscles

Figure 3

Exhalation

trachea

pectoralis
minor

lung

diaphragm

intercostal
muscles

vice versa. This occurs because the flow of blood shifts back and forth between the nostrils in a rhythm that takes approximately one and a half to two hours.[6]

After passing through the nose, the air then flows down past our pharynx, the cavity at the back of our mouth where the nose and mouth are connected, and where swallowing and breathing are coordinated by the pharyngeal plexus (under the control of the lower brain stem). Here the air passes through the lymphoid tissue of the adenoids and tonsils at the back of the nose and throat, where bacteria and viruses are removed. The air then moves past the larynx, which helps the vocal cords use air to produce sound, and then continues downward into the tube of muscle called the trachea, which separates into two bronchi serving the lungs (Figure 4). The trachea and bronchi are lined with mucus-secreting cells that trap pollutants and bacteria. As the air flows through the bronchi, tiny hairlike lashes called cilia massage the mucus and any remaining debris away from the lungs and upward toward the trachea, over the larynx, and finally into the esophagus. When too many particles, chemicals, or clumps of mucus accumulate in the bronchi, they trigger a coughing spasm—a powerful muscle contraction and bronchial constriction which can generate a wind force stronger than a tornado—to expel this toxic material.

In the lungs, the bronchi divide into smaller and smaller branches called bronchioles. The bronchioles, which have muscular walls that can constrict air flow through contraction, end in some 400 million bubble-like sacs called alveoli. It is in the alveoli that the life-giving exchange between oxygen and carbon dioxide occurs—where fresh oxygen enters the circulatory system to be carried throughout the body by hemoglobin molecules in the blood, and where gaseous waste products such as carbon dioxide are returned by the blood for elimination through exhalation.

THE PHASES OF BREATHING

Depending on the demands of what we are doing at the moment (lying down, sitting, walking, running) and on our specific psychological state (peaceful, angry, stressed out, happy), our breath can range from fast to slow and from shallow to deep, emphasizing one or more of the three fundamental phases of the breathing process: *diaphragmatic, thoracic, and clavicular.* In deep breathing, for example—what is often referred to as "the yogic complete breath," all three phases come into play. According to Alan Hymes, M.D., a cardiovascular and thoracic surgeon who is a pioneer in the field of breath research, this form of breathing "is initiated by diaphragmatic contraction, resulting in a slight expansion of the lower ribs and protrusion of the upper abdomen, thus oxygenating the lower lung fields. Then the middle portions of the lungs expand, with outward chest movement, in the thoracic phase as inhalation proceeds further. At the very end of inhalation, still more air is admitted by slightly raising the clavicles, thereby expanding the uppermost tips of the lungs. In sequence, then, each phase of inhalation acts on one particular area of the lungs."[7] As we shall see, no matter what state we may be in, most of us depend mainly on chest and clavicular breathing, and have little experience of diaphragmatic breathing. Thus, we seldom draw air into the deepest areas of our lungs, where most of our blood awaits oxygenation.

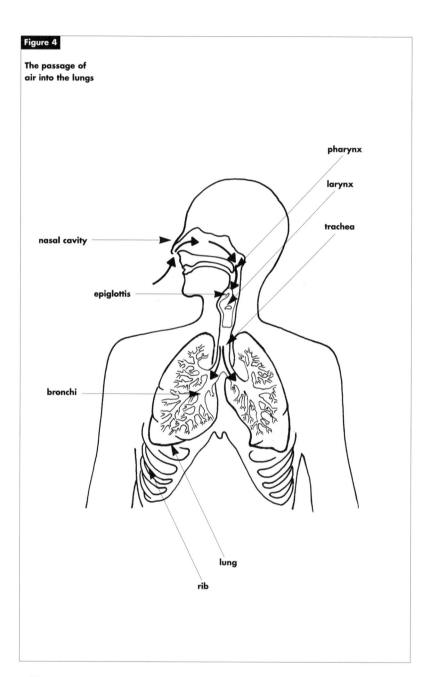

Figure 4

The passage of
air into the lungs

pharynx

larynx

trachea

nasal cavity

epiglottis

bronchi

lung

rib

THE INNER BREATH

Whatever outer form our breath takes, an inner process of breathing also occurs. This process takes place in the cells, which inhale oxygen from the steady stream of hemoglobin flowing throughout the body and exhale carbon dioxide back into this stream. It is in the cells, and more particularly the mitochondria, where the inhaled oxygen helps transform food into biological energy. This transformation occurs when oxygen is combined with carbon (from food) in a slow-burning fire. The energy released from the interaction of oxygen and carbon is transferred to energy storage molecules, called ATP (adenosine triphosphate), which make it available to all the cells of the body. Waste products, such as carbon dioxide, are returned to the venous blood and ultimately to the lungs and back into the atmosphere.

THE RESPIRATORY CENTER

The process of breathing and its relationship to the production of energy in our organism is so fundamental to our survival that nature has given us little direct control over it. Our breathing is thus mostly involuntary, generally controlled by the respiratory center of the autonomic nervous system—especially the vagus nucleus in the medulla oblongata, the nervous tissue at the floor of the fourth ventricle of the brain (Figure 5). The respiratory center, which is located near the occiput (where the spine meets the skull), transmits impulses to nerves in the spinal cord that cause the diaphragm and intercostal muscles to begin the process of inhalation. Branches of the vagus nerve coming from this center sense the stretching of the lungs during inhalation and then automatically inhibit inhalation so that exhalation can take place. The respiratory system is connected to most of the body's sensory nerves; hence any sudden or chronic stimulation coming through any of the senses can have an immediate impact on the force or speed of our breath, or can stop it altogether. Intense beauty, for example, can momentarily "take our breath away," while pain, tension, or stress generally speeds up our breathing and reduces its depth. We can, of

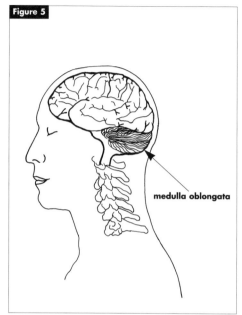

Figure 5

medulla oblongata

course—within limits—intentionally hold our breath, lengthen or reduce our inhalation and exhalation, breathe more deeply, and so on. When we do so, the nerve impulses generated in the cerebral cortex as a result of our intention bypass the respiratory center and travel down the same path used for voluntary muscle control.

Acid/Alkaline Balance

The respiratory center does its work based on the acid/alkaline balance of the blood. The cells in the nucleus of the medulla are sensitive to this balance. From the standpoint of our health, the blood must remain slightly alkaline (pH 7.4). Even tiny deviations from this condition can be dangerous. When the body's chemical activity increases because of physical effort, emotional stress, sensory stimulation, and so on, more carbon dioxide and other acids are produced. This increases the acidity of the blood. To counteract this increase and maintain homeostasis, the respiratory center automatically increases the breath rate. This helps to bring in needed oxygen and to expel excess carbon dioxide. When the body's chemical activity decreases through relaxation or rest, less carbon dioxide is produced and our breathing automatically slows down.[8]

Though we cannot, for the most part, alter the basic chemistry of the respiratory process, we can influence it in a variety of "indirect" ways. One such way is through the relaxation of excessive tension in our postures, movements, and actions. Tension, which involves muscular contraction, produces both lactic acid and carbon dioxide. By reducing chronic tension, we reduce the quantity of these waste products, as well as the work that the body needs to do to counteract them. The relaxation of chronic tension also makes possible the more efficient coordination of the various mechanisms involved in breathing. It is through the harmonious coordination of these mechanisms that we can take in oxygen and expel carbon dioxide with the least possible expenditure of the body's resources.

THE RESPIRATORY MUSCLES

Healthy breathing involves the harmonious interplay not just of the rib muscles, abdominal muscles, and diaphragm, but also of various other muscles throughout the body. These include the extensor muscles of the back, which keep us vertical in relation to gravity, and the psoas muscles, which connect the vertebrae in the lower thoracic and lumbar areas to the pelvis and thigh bones, and are involved in both hip and spinal flexion (Figure 6). Unnecessary tension in the muscles of our shoulders, chest, belly, back, or pelvis—whether it is caused by negative emotions, physical or psychological stress, trauma, injury, or faulty posture—increases the level of carbon dioxide in our blood and interferes with respiratory coordination. It also overstimulates our sensory nerves, which, as we will see later, has an unhealthy influence on our overall functioning.

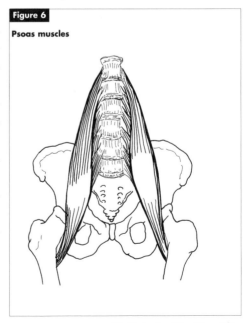

Figure 6

Psoas muscles

The Diaphragm—the "Spiritual Muscle"

Of all the respiratory muscles, the most important from the standpoint of our overall health is the diaphragm. Though few of us make efficient use of this muscle, it nevertheless lies at the foundation of healthy breathing. Shaped like a large dome, the diaphragm functions as both the floor of the chest cavity and the ceiling of the abdominal cavity (Figure 7). It is penetrated by—and can affect—several important structures, including the esophagus, which carries food to the stomach; the aorta, which carries blood from the heart to the arteries of all the limbs and organs except the lungs; the vena cava, the central vein that carries venous blood from the various parts of the body back to the heart; and various nerves including the vagus nerve, which descends from the medulla oblongata and branches to the various internal organs.

Although breathing can continue even if the diaphragm stops functioning, it is the rhythmical contraction and relaxation of the diaphragm that animates our breath and plays an important role in promoting physical and psychological health. When we inhale, the diaphragm normally contracts. This pulls the top of its dome downward toward the abdominal organs, while the various chest muscles expand the rib cage slightly outward and upward. This pumplike motion creates a partial vacuum, which, as we know, draws air into the lungs. When we inhale fully, the diaphragm can double or even triple its range of movement and actually massage—directly in some cases, indirectly in others—the stomach, liver, pancreas, intestines, and kidneys, promoting intestinal movement, blood and lymph flow, and the absorption of nutrients.

Even a slight increase in the diaphragm's movement downward not only has a beneficial impact on our internal organs, but also brings about a large increase in the air volume of the lungs. For every additional millimeter the diaphragm expands, the volume of air in our lungs increases by some 250 to 300 milliliters. Research done in mainland China demonstrates that novices working with deep breathing can learn to increase the downward movement of their diaphragms by an average of four millimeters in six to 12 months. They are thus able to increase the volume of air in their lungs by more than 1,000 milliliters—in a year or less.[9]

At maximum inhalation, the muscles of the abdomen naturally contract to counterbalance the movement of the diaphragm downward and help limit the further expansion of the lungs. As exhalation begins, the diaphragm relaxes upward, its elasticity helping to expel used air from the lungs. When we exhale completely, the diaphragm projects firmly up against the heart and lungs, giving these organs life and support. For Taoist master Mantak Chia, the diaphragm is nothing less than *a spiritual muscle.* "Lifting the heart and fanning the fires of digestion and metabolism, the diaphragm muscle plays a largely unheralded role in maintaining our health, vitality, and well-being."[10]

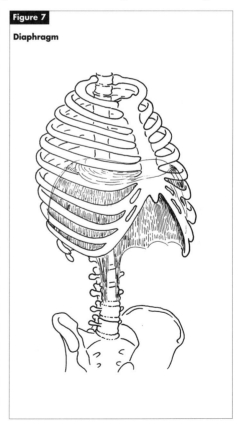

Figure 7

Diaphragm

Restrictive Influences on the Diaphragm

Unfortunately, most of us do not experience the full benefit of this "spiritual muscle." There are two major reasons for this. First, the movement of the diaphragm is adversely influenced by the sympathetic nervous system as a result of the chronic stress, fear, and negativity in our lives (I will discuss the sympathetic nervous system in more detail in the next chapter). Second, it is also adversely influenced by unnecessary tension in our muscles, tendons, and ligaments, as well as by the faulty configurations of our skeletal structure. In understanding this second point, it is useful to know something about how and where the diaphragm actually attaches to the skeletal structure. Though most of the body's muscles are attached to two different bones—one fixed, called the "origin," and one which moves as a result of muscle contraction, called the "insert"—the diaphragm is not attached in this way. The diaphragm is fixed to the inside of the lower ribs as well as to the lumbar spine, close to the psoas muscles, but it does not "insert" to any bone. Rather, it inserts to its own central tendon, which lies just under the heart (Figure 8). The diaphragm

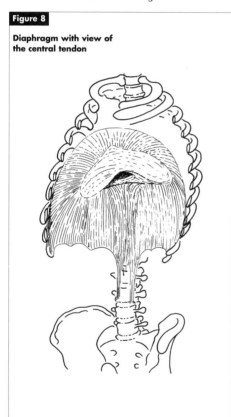

Figure 8

Diaphragm with view of the central tendon

is thus influenced by the health and mobility of the spine and pelvis, and their associated muscles, and these in turn are influenced not just by our habitual postures, but also by our emotions and attitudes.

One of the most adverse influences on the movement of the diaphragm is the unnecessary tension that many of us carry in our abdominal muscles and internal organs. Most of these tensions are the result of chronic stress, repressed emotions, and excessive negativity, but they also can be caused by the prevailing image of the hard, flat belly that we find in fashion magazines and fitness centers. When the belly is overly contracted it resists the downward movement of the diaphragm. When this occurs, the diaphragm's central tendon replaces the rib cage and spine as the diaphragm's fixed point, and the contraction of the diaphragm during inhalation causes excessive elevation of the ribs.

Compensating for a Poorly Functioning Diaphragm

To attempt to compensate for decreased lung space resulting from a contracted belly and a poorly functioning diaphragm—especially in times of physical or psychological stress (when more energy is needed)—we either have to breathe faster (which may result in hyperventilation and the emergence of the "fight or flight reflex") or we have to increase the expansion of the thoracic cage and raise the clavicles. Because the thoracic cage and clavicles are relatively rigid, however, this further expansion requires the expenditure of extra muscular effort and energy, and ultimately results in less oxygen being taken in during each breath.

If someone were to ask us to take a deep breath, most of us would make a big effort to suck in our belly, expand our upper chest, and raise our shoulders—a not-so-funny caricature of "chest breathing"—the way most of us breathe most of the time (Figure 9). Such an effort, however, results in a shallow breath, not a deep one. As we shall see more clearly in later chapters, a deep inhalation requires the expansion of the abdomen outward,

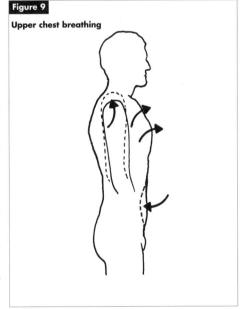

Figure 9

Upper chest breathing

which helps the diaphragm move further downward and allows the bottom of the lungs to expand more completely. Though it is true that raising the shoulders reduces the weight on the ribs beneath and allows the lungs to expand further at the top, the potential volume at the top of the lungs is much smaller than the potential volume at the bottom. Expanding the top of the chest and raising the shoulders may be an effective emergency measure to take in more air for those of us with little elasticity in our diaphragm, rib cage, and belly, or who have asthma or emphysema, but for most of us it only further entrenches our bad breathing habits and undermines our health and vitality.

THE HARMFUL EFFECTS OF BAD BREATHING HABITS

Breathing based on such habits—habits in which the diaphragm is unable to extend through its full range and activate and support the rhythmical movement of the abdominal muscles, organs, and tissues— has many harmful effects on the organism. It reduces the efficiency of our lungs and thus the amount of oxygen available to our cells. It necessitates that we take from two to four times as many breaths as we would with natural, abdominal breathing, and thus increases energy expenditure through higher breath and heart rates. It retards venous blood flow, which carries metabolic wastes from the cells to the kidneys and lungs where they can be excreted before they do harm to the organism. (In this regard, it is important to realize that 70 percent of the body's waste products are eliminated through the lungs, while the rest are eliminated through the urine, feces, and skin.) It retards the functioning of the lymphatic system, whose job it is to trap and destroy viral and bacterial invaders, and thus gives these invaders more time to cause disease. It also reduces the amount of digestive juices, including the enzyme pepsin, available for the digestive process, and slows down the process of peristalsis in the small and large intestines. This causes toxins to pile up and fester throughout the digestive tract. In short, such breathing weakens and disharmonizes the functioning of almost every major system in the body and makes us more susceptible to chronic and acute illnesses and "dis-eases" of all kinds: infections, constipation, respiratory illnesses, digestive problems, ulcers, depression, sexual disorders, sleep disorders, fatigue, headaches, poor blood circulation, premature aging, and so on. Many researchers even believe that our bad breathing habits also contribute to life-threatening diseases such as cancer and heart disease.

Through the gentle, natural practices in this book, however, we can begin to discover the power of natural breathing to counteract these habits and support the overall health, vitality, and well-being that is our birthright.

PRACTICE

The first step to working with your breath is to be clear in your mind about the actual mechanics, the physiological "laws," of natural breathing. This mental clarity will help you experience the breathing process both more directly and more accurately. The next step is to deepen your awareness of your own particular breathing patterns. For your first exercise, read this chapter again; as you read, visualize and sense in yourself the various mechanisms being discussed. Don't try to change anything; just see what you can learn about your own particular breathing process. In the next chapter you'll have an opportunity to go more deeply into the process of self-sensing and its relationship to your breath and health.

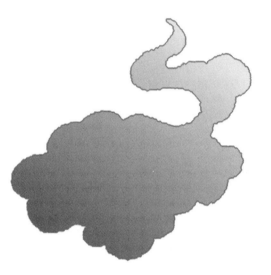

BREATH, EMOTIONS, AND THE ART OF SELF-SENSING

... the work with breathing starts
with sensing the inner atmosphere
of our organism—
the basic emotional stance we take
toward ourselves and the world.

The integration of natural breathing into our lives begins with learning how to sense ourselves more completely and accurately—to consciously occupy our bodies. It is through conscious embodiment, the whole sensation of ourselves, that we can awaken to higher levels of organic intelligence, to the "wisdom" of the body. Though we all have the potential to sense our bodies in their entirety, the sensory image we have of ourselves is generally fragmentary and filled with distortions. What's more, the body we think we know so well is in large part a "historical" body— a body shaped by the past, by the results of our long-forgotten physical and emotional responses to the conditions of our early lives. It is also, of course, shaped by the present, especially by our lack of sensory awareness.

THE WORK OF SENSORY AWARENESS

The term "sensory awareness" first became popular in America in the late 1960s, mainly through the work of Charlotte Selver (who had been giving workshops in America since 1938) and Charles Brooks, two of the pioneers in the human potential movement.[11] Their work was concerned in large part with the effort to discover through sensation what is natural in our functioning, and what is conditioned; what opens us to the reality of the present moment, and what closes us. It is, of course, questions such as these—and the answers that we can we experience in our own individual lives—that are crucial to our health, well-being, and inner growth. Enriched by the psychophysical experiments of Esalen Institute, in Big Sur, California, and the entry of various Asian spiritual traditions into America in the 1960s and 1970s—especially traditions such as Zen Buddhism, Tibetan Buddhism, and Taoism—the work of sensory awareness demonstrated a new, more fundamental way of relating to ourselves and our energies.

Though the work of sensory awareness begins with our inner and outer senses, it reaches far beyond them into the very meaning of consciousness. Anyone who seriously undertakes this work will quickly discover two remarkable facts. First, that we generally live our lives in a state of "somatic amnesia"—a state in which we are mostly oblivious to the rich, informative sensation of our bodies. What awareness we do have of our bodies is not only filled with enormous gaps, but is often just plain wrong, as physical therapists, body workers, and others are quick to point out. Second, that this somatic amnesia is closely related to our "emotional amnesia," our frequent inability to feel the emotions and attitudes that are actually motivating our behavior. The gaps in the overall sensation of our bodies are not merely gaps in our bodily awareness; they also represent gaps in our mental and emotional awareness.

As a result of our lack of "integral awareness," awareness that encompasses our entire being, we have lost touch not only with the gracefulness in action that is our birthright, but, even more importantly, with the extraordinary capabilities of the human organism to sense itself from the inside and to learn new and better ways of functioning through this sensation. Even many of us involved in physical fitness and martial arts have little conscious contact with our bodies, approaching them not through ever-deepening organic awareness but rather through memory, willfulness, coercion, and repetition. The slogan "no pain, no gain" is an extreme example of this approach.

THE WORLD IN THE BODY

From the perspective of Taoism, as well as of Chinese medicine, this lack of integral awareness is harmful to our health. It also deprives us of the vision, the perspective, we need for psychological or spiritual evolution. For the Taoist, the statement "as above, so below" is one of the fundamental truths of life. The body (including the brain) is a microcosm of the universe, and operates under the same laws. Not only is the body "in the world," but the world is "in the body"—especially the *conscious body*. For those who can be sensitive, who can learn how to sense themselves impartially, the rich landscape of the outer world—the rivers, lakes, oceans, tides, fields, mountains, deserts, caves, forests, and so on—has direct counterparts in the inner world of the body. The energetic and material qualities of the outer world—represented in Taoism by "the five elements": fire, earth, metal, water, and wood—manifest in the body as the network of primary organs: the heart, spleen, lungs, kidneys, and liver. And the atmospheric movements of matter and energy that we call "weather"—wind, rain, storm, warmth, cold, dampness, dryness, and so on—have their obvious counterparts in the inner atmosphere of our emotions. Likewise, the cosmic metabolism of the outer world—the conservation, transformation, and use of the energies of the earth, atmosphere, sun, moon, and stars—has its counterpart in the metabolism of our inner world, in the movement and transformation of food, air, and energy. To begin to sense the interrelationships and rhythms of the various functions of one's own body—of one's skin, muscles, bones, organs, tissues, nerves, fluids, hormones, emotions, and thoughts—is to experience the energies and laws of life itself. As Lao Tzu says: "Without leaving his house, he knows the whole world. Without looking out of his window, he sees the ways of heaven."

Whether or not we agree with this vision of our organism as a microcosm of the universe, the work of self-sensing will quickly show us that the rhythms of breathing—of inhalation and exhalation—lie at the heart of our physical, emotional, and spiritual lives. We will see that it is through the sensory experience of these rhythms that we can awaken our inner sensitivity and awareness and begin to open ourselves to our inner healing powers—the creative power of nature itself. But for this to occur, our breathing must change from "normal" to "natural"; it must become free from the unconscious motivations and constraints of our self-image.

PERCEPTUAL REEDUCATION AND WHOLENESS

Our faulty patterns of breathing have developed over many years and are tied in closely with our self-image, with our individual patterns of illusion, avoidance, and forgetfulness. As a result, correcting them is not just a matter of applying the right techniques. Nor is it just a matter of going to a physical therapist or other body work practitioner to learn proper breathing mechanics, as we might go to an auto mechanic to fix a faulty carburetor or muffler. It is, rather, a matter of *perceptual reeducation,* of learning how to experience ourselves in an entirely new way, and from an entirely new perspective.

The etymology of the verb *to heal* is related to the verb *to make whole.* To become whole, however, it is first necessary, as Gurdjieff says, to *know that I am not whole*—to sense my dis-ease, to actually see and come to terms with my imbalance, my fragmentation, my illusions, my contradictions, and my incomplete sensation of myself. Self-healing thus begins with awareness and acceptance of "what is," of the living reality of my psychosomatic structure—the ways in which my thoughts, emotions, and sensations interact with my chemistry, physiology, and psychology. The awareness of "what is," however, is not something I can bring about by force. It depends on discovering a dimension in myself of inner quiet, of inner clarity—a clear, uncolored lens through which I can observe myself without any judgment, criticism, or analysis. This inner clarity, which Gurdjieff calls "presence," is both a precondition and a result of work with sensation and breath.

THE IMPORTANCE OF FOLLOWING THE BREATH

One of the very first steps of this work, therefore—a step that on no account must be skipped—is to learn how to "follow," to sense, the movements of our breath without interfering with them or trying to change them in any way. This work of following—which is left out of many teachings and therapies—provides the stable foundation of inner perception required for sensing the various mechanisms involved in breathing, as well as observing the physical, emotional, and mental forces acting on them. As Ilse Middendorf, one of the great pioneers in breath therapy, has pointed out, it is by perceiving our breath as it comes and goes that we discover an opening into our own unconscious life, and bring about a conscious expansion into the whole of ourselves.[12] It is my experience that this expansion of awareness, this conscious "welcoming" of everything that we are, lies at the heart of deep, inner quiet and relaxation—an organic release from the stranglehold of our self-image, and from the excessive tension, stress, and negativity in our inner and outer lives. It is this welcoming that is the foundation of wholeness, of real health.

LISTENING TO THE BODY

Learning how to observe the mechanisms involved in breathing, as well as the various physical, emotional, and mental forces acting on them, depends in large part on learning how to sense ourselves, to listen to ourselves, to expand our attention to include the sensory impressions constantly arising in our organism. Though it sometimes happens spontaneously, listening to our bodies in the midst of action is relatively rare. It demands that we learn how to be attentive in two directions at once: outwardly toward the conditions and actions of our outer lives, and inwardly toward the thoughts, emotions, and sensations of our inner lives. For it is only when we can be aware of both our inner and outer worlds *at the same time,* that we can go beyond the beliefs of our self-image and experience the real forces at work in us.

Learning how to "listen" to the continual flow of information that our body gives us is not easy. It demands that we live not in our dreams and imagination, but rather in the reality of the present moment. As psychoanalyst Rollo May points out, "In our society it often requires considerable effort to listen to the body—an effort of sustained 'openness' to whatever cues may be coming from one's body." May was confronted with the necessity of listening to his own body when, in the 1940s, he discovered that he had tuberculosis. At the time, "the only cure was bed rest and carefully graduated exercise ... I found that listening to my body was of critical importance in my cure. When I could be sensitive to my body, 'hear' that I was fatigued and needed to rest more, or sense that my body was strong enough for me to increase my exercise, I got better. And when I found awareness of my body blocked off ... I got worse."[13]

SELF-SENSING—THE BEGINNING OF SELF-KNOWLEDGE AND SELF-TRANSFORMATION

Self-sensing brings us a more genuine relationship with ourselves, and with our own real needs, since it reveals how we are actually responding to the inner and outer circumstances of our lives. It also has a direct impact on our nervous system, helping to bring about the changes necessary for harmonious functioning and development. In understanding how these changes take place, it is important to realize that the human brain is composed of some 100 billion neurons, each of which "touches" approximately 10,000 other neurons. The main function of these neurons is to connect distant parts of the organism with one other, so that the organism can function as an integrated whole in carrying out its actions. The majority of these neurons are associated, directly or indirectly, with some kind of motion. And this motion depends on information, on sensory feedback, from both inside and outside of the organism. From the perspective of science, then, the main function of the brain is the correlation of our actions with the sensory data upon which these actions depend.

As we begin to sense ourselves more completely, we will experience firsthand how the correlation between our actions and our senses enters into almost every aspect of our lives. We will see, for example, how the motor cortex—the part of the brain that controls our voluntary muscular system and is thus involved in every intentional movement we make—depends on the sensory cortex to provide continuing feedback for its operations. The sensory cortex gets its information not only from the external senses, such as sight, smell, hearing, and touch, but also from our various internal senses. Our kinesthetic sensations, for example, come from stretch receptors in the muscles, joints, tendons, and ligaments, and our organic sensations come from the various nerve receptors in our organs, tissues, and skin. It is only when the motor cortex has the most complete, accurate information available to it from the sensory cortex that it can execute our intentions in the most efficient, balanced, and healthy way possible. Self-sensing helps provide this information.

Through self-sensing we not only learn about the subtle, constantly changing needs of our bodies, but we also begin to learn about the impact of our emotions on our breath, and thus on our health and well-being. By "listening" to the sensation of our body, especially our breathing, not only when we are in quiet circumstances but also when we are in the middle of difficult situations in our lives, we experience connections between parts of ourselves that ordinarily escape our attention. By sensing the way our breathing changes in relation to changing circumstances, as well as by sensing the attitudes, tensions, postures, and emotions that arise in these same conditions, we begin to learn, with exacting detail, about the intimate relationship of our breath to our overall sense of ourselves. This new, direct knowledge of ourselves in action gives our brain and nervous system the knowledge and perspective it needs to help free us from our habitual psychophysical patterns of action and reaction. Self-sensing helps create new connections between existing neurons in the brain and nervous system. These new connections help increase our overall awareness, and promote greater sensitivity and flexibility in our perception and behavior.

THE THREE KINDS OF BREATH

As we begin this work of self-sensing, we may observe three kinds of breath in our life. First, and most common, is the *balanced breath,* which more or less balances inhalation and exhalation, yang and yin, the sympathetic nervous system and the parasympathetic nervous system. This breath, however shallow or full, reflects the automatic, mostly unconscious equilibrium of our lives. Second, is the *cleansing breath,* which emphasizes exhalation over inhalation. This breath sometimes takes place spontaneously as a sigh or moan when we are physically or emotionally overloaded with toxins or tensions. The long exhalation helps us to relax and to rid the body of these toxins, especially carbon dioxide. Third, is the *energizing breath,* which emphasizes inhalation over exhalation. This breath sometimes takes place spontaneously as a yawn when we are tired or bored. The long, deep inhalation brings us more oxygen and thus more energy, and helps motivate us to take action.

THE QUALITY OF OUR BREATHING

The quality of our inhalation and exhalation reveals a great deal about our stance toward life. We may observe, for example, how the extent and comfort of our inhalation reflects our readiness and ability to embrace life at that moment, and how the extent and comfort of our exhalation reflects our readiness and ability to let go, to trust something other than the accouterments of our self-image. We may notice how during fear or other strong negative emotions we restrict the flow of breath by contracting various parts of our body in order to reduce the energy available for feeling, and how during more pleasant emotions we increase the flow and duration of breath to take in more energy and thus to feel more.

Hyperventilation and Anxiety

In sensing the "quality" of our breath, many of us may also notice that even at rest we breathe faster than the "average" rate of 12 to 14 times a minute (a rate which is already faster than it needs to be). In fact, many of us, without knowing it, habitually "hyperventilate"—that is, we take quick, shallow breaths from the top of our chest. These quick, shallow breaths sharply reduce the level of carbon dioxide in our blood. This reduced level of carbon dioxide causes the arteries, including the carotid artery going to the brain, to constrict, thus reducing the flow of blood throughout the body. When this occurs, no matter how much oxygen we may breathe into our lungs, our brain and body will experience a shortage of oxygen. The lack of oxygen switches on the sympathetic nervous system—our "fight or flight" reflex—which makes us tense, anxious, and irritable. It also reduces our ability to think clearly, and tends to put us at the mercy of obsessive thoughts and images. Some researchers believe that hyperventilation can actually magnify our psychological problems and conflicts, and that chronic hyperventilation is intimately bound up with our anxieties, apprehensions, and fears.[14]

The Emotional Topography of Our Breath

As our ability to sense ourselves grows, we will begin to receive many precise impressions of the interrelationships of our emotions and breath, and their impact on our overall sensation of ourselves. We may see, for example, how anger is associated with shallow inhalations, strong exhalations, and tension throughout the body—especially in the neck, jaw, chest, and hands. We may see how fear is associated with rapid, shallow, and irregular breaths, and the sensation of a tight knot in the lower abdomen. We may see how grief or sorrow is associated with a kind of spasmodic, sobbing, superficial breath, and a hollow, empty feeling in the belly. We may see how impatience is associated with short, jerky, uncoordinated breaths, and tension in the front of the chest, as though our hearts were leaping ahead of us. We may see how guilt or self-judgment is associated with a restricted, suffocating breath, and an overall sensation of being weighed down. And we may see how boredom is associated with a shallow, lifeless breath, and little sensation anywhere in ourselves. We may also notice how feelings such as love, compassion, kindness, and wonder are associated with deep, comfortable breathing, and an open, energized, receptive feeling throughout the entire body. Each of us, of course, will discover variations in his or her own physical and emotional topography.

"Every State of Mind is a State of Our Immune System"

Such observations are important not only from the standpoint of self-knowledge, but also from the standpoint of our health and well-being. Though many traditions and teachings besides Taoism speak of the intimate relationship of mind and body—the way in which our thoughts, emotions, and body influence one another—it is only recently in the West that science has begun to uncover the underlying chemistry of this relationship. At a lecture I attended in April 1995, at the California Pacific Medical Center in San Francisco, Candace Pert, Ph.D., a world-renown pioneer in the area of neuroscience, stated that the evidence now shows that "every state of mind is a state of our immune system."

She spoke dramatically about how "messenger molecules" called "neuropeptides" carry information from brain to body and body to brain to direct energy in the organism. She asserted that these neuropeptides, which include the chemicals known as endorphins, are the "biochemical correlates of emotions," and can have a powerful influence on our health.[15] When someone asked Pert how she would use this knowledge if she had to undergo serious surgery, she replied that she would spend time with the surgeon to understand the operation—to know which organs and procedures would be involved. She suggested that this understanding, combined with visualization of the healing process, could help release those neuropeptides necessary to promote healing.

Self-knowledge Can Improve Our Health

From both the Taoist and scientific perspectives, it is clear that in the right context self-knowledge can have a powerful and beneficial influence on our immune system. But to acquire this knowledge in a way that is useful to us, to gain a deep understanding of the various mental, emotional, and physical forces acting on our health and well-being, we need to learn how to sense our bodies—our muscles, organs, bones, tissues, and so on—more impartially. We need to learn how to take "sensory snapshots" of our organic functioning. As we do, we will begin to observe the various habits of our psychophysical structure, along with the physiological principles that give these habits their power to influence our health. We will begin to see the particular ways that we respond mentally and emotionally to the various stresses of our lives, to the threats and demands that we often unconsciously perceive in relation to new or changing circumstances. This is important, since it is now believed that stress-related disorders account—either directly or indirectly—for 50 to 80 percent of all illnesses. Such disorders include chronic colds, hypertension, heart disease, high blood pressure, ulcers, irritable bowel syndrome, depression, arthritis, insomnia, certain types of cancer, and many more.

One of the ways that stress undermines our health is by increasing the production of the hormone cortisol, which in turn suppresses our immune system. A study published in the early 1990s in *The New England Journal of Medicine* found, for instance, that healthy participants who were given nose drops containing a cold virus were susceptible to the virus in direct relationship to the degree of emotional stress they were experiencing at the time. Other studies have shown that stress—and the fear and anxiety often associated with it—can cause autoimmune diseases such as multiple sclerosis and rheumatoid arthritis to worsen.[16] Through learning how to sense ourselves more clearly, however, we will begin to understand that it is not always stress itself that is the problem—a certain amount of stress can actually be beneficial to our health—*but rather the habitual ways in which we respond to stress.* It is here that our emotions play a major role.

EMOTIONS AND THE AUTONOMIC NERVOUS SYSTEM

Through self-sensing we will begin to experience for ourselves the relationship between our emotions and the so-called autonomic nervous system, which controls the smooth muscles and the glands. This system works either to excite or inhibit certain internal and external actions and secretions. As we learn how to sense the physiological effects of fear, anger, and anxiety in ourselves, for example, we will begin to understand experientially how they are bound up with the sympathetic branch of the autonomic nervous system, which readies the body for "fight or flight" action. The sympathetic system acts in "sympathy" with our emotions, particularly those related to fear, danger, and excitement. Some signs that this system is turned on include sweating, dry mouth, and other forms of "arousal." This system, with neurons located mainly in the chest and midback regions of the spine, communicates with the rest of the body by transmitting impulses from the brain through chains of sympathetic ganglia running down both sides of the spine. From the ganglia, nerve fibers carry impulses to the various internal organs. These nerve impulses decrease movement in the digestive organs, increase heart rate and blood pressure, constrict blood vessels, dilate (open up) airways in the lungs, release sugar stored in the liver, and flood the body with adrenaline and norepinephrine from the adrenal glands, so that more blood and energy are available for action.

The Survival Value of Negative Emotions

As troublesome as they are in our lives, it is clear—at least sometimes—that what we call "negative emotions" have important "survival" value. Many of our negative emotions are simply signals that something has gone wrong in our lives or that some action is necessary to avoid a potential problem. A student's anxiety about an upcoming exam, or an executive's anxiety about a financial report that is due the next day, can play a beneficial role in stimulating appropriate preparation, as long as the anxiety does not become so excessive that it causes fear and a lack of concentration. A woman's anger toward a man who physically or psychologically abuses her may motivate her to leave the relationship or to find a healthier relationship with someone else, as long as it doesn't become so strong that she becomes violent. A mother's anger toward a teenage daughter who stays out all night may be what is necessary to motivate both mother and daughter to try to communicate with each other in a new way. Our lives are filled with many examples of how our so-called negative emotions, as long as they do not become excessive, can provide important information about what is happening in our lives—information that can help us take intelligent actions on behalf of ourselves and others.

Unfortunately, many of our negative emotions seem to quickly reach a point where they have no apparent solution, and we frequently find ourselves unable to learn anything from them or to do anything about them. These emotions leave us with pounding hearts, contracted muscles, poor digestion, constipation, tension, and so on. Over time, these conditions can become chronic and can consume the energy we need for healing and for inner growth. Once these conditions become habitual, the parasympathetic branch of the autonomic nervous system, designed to put the brakes on the sympathetic nervous system, will have little power to bring about more than temporary relief—unless we can learn how to consciously turn it on for longer periods of time.

Learning to Turn On the Parasympathetic Nervous System

To learn how to turn on the parasympathetic nervous system, it is useful to know something about its organization. The neurons for this system reside mainly in certain cranial nerves, such as the vagus nerve, coming from the brain stem, and in the lower-back region of the spine. The parasympathetic ganglia do not run down the spine, but instead are located near the organs that they influence. Impulses coming from these ganglia reduce the heart rate, dilate the blood vessels, increase digestive peristalsis, and constrict the air passages in the lungs, and thus help the body slow down and restore itself.

How can we intentionally turn on this system, our relaxation response, without the outside help of psychologists, massage therapists, and so on? The key is our *attention*. We know from experience that when we are tense or "stressed out" our attention—directed by the sympathetic nervous system—automatically focuses on the supposed cause of our tension, the compulsive thoughts and feelings that arise in relation to it, or the particular unpleasant physical symptoms we are experiencing. As a result, our experience of ourselves becomes so narrow that we cannot even imagine an alternative. To learn how to relax in such situations, we need to learn how to work actively with our attention, to widen it to include the parts of ourselves that are not in the grip of the negativity we are experiencing. One of the most effective ways to accomplish this is through self-sensing. According to Ernest Rossi, a pioneer in the field of mind/body interaction, "You simply close your eyes and tune into the parts of your body that are most comfortable. When you locate the comfort you simply enjoy it and allow it to deepen and spread throughout your body all by itself. Comfort is more than just a word or a lazy state. Really going deeply into comfort means that you have turned on your parasympathetic system—your natural relaxation response."[17] As we shall see later, natural breathing plays an important role in learning how to go "deeply into comfort," and thus in learning how to use our awareness to harmonize the aggressive and restorative functions of our nervous system.[18] What's more, since natural breathing massages our internal organs and relaxes our lower back, it has a beneficial influence on the parasympathetic nerves and ganglia in these areas.

Unfortunately, most of us are not very good at sensing ourselves and have little awareness of the extent to which our perception and behavior are conditioned by emotions such as fear, anger, and anxiety. We have become so accustomed to high levels of stress and negativity in our lives that we take it as "normal," not realizing the tremendous toll it takes on our health and vitality. The noise produced by this stress makes it almost impossible to hear the quiet, ever-present intelligence of our own bodies. Unable to experience this inner intelligence, we exacerbate our situation by seeking quick relief through excessive stimulation of some kind—alcohol, drugs, tobacco, caffeine, food, sex, television, and so on. Sometimes, when we wake up for a moment to the senselessness of our situation, we may try to deal rationally with the stresses we face. But our minds by themselves have little power to "figure out" effective solutions—especially in an "information society" that floods our consciousness with negative news and images from around the world. The end result is the accumulation of more and more tension, a sense of helplessness, and the eventual appearance of various chronic symptoms and ailments in our lives—many of which are not just the result of stresses we face, but also of the way we try to escape them.

Coping with the Effects of Stress Is Not the Solution

Unable to figure out effective solutions to the many stresses in our lives, we have over time learned various ways to "cope" with their effects on us instead. Some of us, for example, simply vent our negative emotions, especially anger, on others, believing that this is good for us. Recent studies suggest, however, that venting our anger causes us to get more angry, not less, and thus increases our health risks.[19] What's more, such an action simply spreads our negativity to others, adding to their own problems.

The expression of negative emotions, however, is probably not nearly as prevalent as finding ways to avoid experiencing them. As children, some of us learned how to use fantasy and repression to shut ourselves off from the painful feelings of contradiction that we felt when our parents did not seem to accept us as we were, but rather demanded that we "grow up" according to their image. As adults, many of us have learned how to "swallow" our negative emotions and take refuge in what we consider to be our more positive ones. We have learned how to suppress our negative emotions in order to function in what we believe to be a reasonable way based on our self-image. But we know by the scientific law of conservation of energy that the neurochemical energy of these emotions cannot be destroyed—it can only be transformed. And we also know, if we look carefully, that this energy is often transformed into kinetic or mechanical energy that acts, without our awareness, on the nerves, tissues, structures, and movements of our bodies.

The repression or suppression of emotions manifests itself not only in our postures and movements, but also in tensions buried deep in our bodies, tensions that consume our energy and undermine our physical and psychological health. By learning how to sense these tensions in ourselves, we will eventually come face-to-face with our mostly unconscious emotions of anger, worry, fear, anxiety, and so on. The goal is not to get rid of these so-called negative emotions—this would be both impossible and undesirable—but rather to find the courage to experience them fully, to open them to the transformative light of impartial awareness. From the Taoist perspective, when we become fully aware of our negative emotions without amplifying them or trying to defend ourselves against them, the neurochemical energy they activate in us can be transformed into the pure energy of vitality. As the Taoists might say, "clouds, rain, and lightening are as necessary to our environment as sunshine and calm. Without a harmonious balance of both kinds of weather, nature would become barren." It is through our breath, especially through natural breathing, that we can begin to discover this dynamic harmony in ourselves. It is through deep, comfortable, natural breathing that we can begin to activate the parasympathetic nervous system and thus the process of healing—of becoming whole again.

THE IMPORTANCE OF "EFFORTLESS EFFORT"

As we've seen, the work with breathing starts with sensing the *inner* atmosphere of our organism—the basic emotional stance we take toward ourselves and the world. When I first began to work seriously with my breath in order to come into more direct touch with myself, however, I quickly saw that most of my "efforts" were based on force, on will power, not on skill and sensitivity, and that instead of working *with* the laws of natural breathing, I was working *against* them. In short, I was using my sympathetic nervous system to try to turn on my parasympathetic system. The more I "tried" to breathe naturally, the more tension I created in myself. This was an important discovery for me, because it demonstrated the fundamental way in which I undermined my efforts in almost every area of my life. I had learned about the importance of "effortless effort" from my various teachers—the importance of acting not just from *doing* but also from *being*, from a deep inner sensitivity to my situation—but it wasn't until I started working in depth with the inner sensation of my body that I began to integrate my understanding of the physiological and biochemical reasons for this approach with the actual practice of it.

As I went deeper into the meaning of effortless effort, I began to understand through self-sensing that my usual efforts—often driven by unseen attitudes and emotions—brought with them unnecessary muscular tension, which not only wasted my energy but also flooded my body with excessive adrenaline and metabolic wastes. Tension creates heat, and my efforts "heated me up," increasing my heart and breath rates. What's more, this unnecessary tension caused my sensory system to go on alert, sending distress signals to my brain. The more tension I had, the busier my brain become in trying to deal with it. The busier my brain became in dealing with it, the more trouble I had focusing on other matters of importance in my life.

As we begin to learn how to sense ourselves—especially in relation to our breathing—we will quickly see that the sensation of intense effort in the many areas of our lives often signals a "wrong" relationship not only to what we are doing, but, perhaps more importantly, to ourselves. It is not wrong in any moral or ethical way, but simply because it is counterproductive—it goes against the laws of harmonious functioning. Wrong effort constricts our breathing, cuts us off from our own energy, and produces actions that we did not intend. As Moshe Feldenkrais has pointed out, "the sensation of effort is the subjective feeling of wasted movement ... of other actions being enacted besides the one intended."[20] It is clear to me today that as we learn to sense ourselves more completely and impartially, we free up the inner intelligence of our minds and bodies to learn new, better ways to accomplish our aims and promote health in our lives.

"The Law of Least Effort"

To understand how this is possible, it is important to understand that the brain learns and performs best when we use the least possible effort to accomplish a given task. For thousands of years, Taoist masters have emphasized this principle through their advice to use no more than 60 or 70 percent of our capacity in carrying out physical or spiritual practices. The Weber-Fechner psychophysical law demonstrates one reason why this is so important, since it states that the "senses are organized to take notice of differences between two stimuli rather than the absolute intensity of a stimulus."[21] When we try hard "to do" something, when we use unnecessary force to accomplish our goals, our whole body generally ends up becoming tense. This tension makes it more difficult for our brain and nervous systems to discern the subtle sensory impressions necessary to help carry out our intention in the most creative way possible.

The "law of least effort" is not, however, a license for laziness. Our health, well-being, and inner growth all require a dynamic balance of tension and relaxation, of yang and yin. They depend on the ability to know through our inner and outer senses what is necessary and what is not in our efforts and actions. To sense ourselves clearly, we need to be able to experience a part or dimension of ourselves that is quiet, comfortable, and free of unnecessary tension. It is the sensation of subtle impressions coming from this more relaxed place in ourselves that allows us to observe and release the unnecessary tension in other parts of ourselves. In short, effective action requires relaxation. But this relaxation should not be a "collapse" of either our body or our awareness. It is more like the "vigilant relaxation" of a cat. Vigilant relaxation makes it possible to manifest the appropriate degree of contraction—the life-giving tension called "tonus"—in any given situation.

THE POWER OF PERCEPTUAL FREEDOM

There are many obvious reasons for learning how to relax unnecessary tension, but one that is often overlooked is that such relaxation frees the brain to notice and respond to a broader, more-subtle spectrum of data and impressions. It is this increase in "perceptual freedom" that can be one of our major contributions to promoting good health in ourselves, since it allows the brain and other systems of the body to make maximum use of their powers in discerning problems and responding appropriately. The hormones, enzymes, endorphins, T-cells, and neuropeptides being produced by the brain and body change dramatically in relation to our ability to perceive in new ways. To be able to perceive in new ways means that our energies are not locked into old patterns, but are free to respond to the actual needs and possibilities of the moment.

There is a wonderful Taoist story that illustrates the importance of perceptual freedom. A man was plodding along a dusty road carrying a long pole on his shoulder with most of his possessions hanging from the ends of the pole. The driver of a horse-drawn wagon saw the man and offered him a ride in the back of the wagon. The man gratefully accepted. As they moved along the bumpy road, the driver heard loud crashes coming from the back of the wagon. When he looked back he noticed that the man was stumbling about with the heavy pole still on his shoulder, bumping into the sides of the wagon. "Why don't you put down the pole and relax a bit," the driver suggested. "I don't want to add any more weight to your already heavy wagon," the man replied sincerely, trying very hard to keep his balance.

Anyone who has studied martial arts, tai chi, dance, and so on knows that the body is capable of remarkable intelligence, sensitivity, and action when we are able to rid ourselves of unnecessary tension. There is the legend of the tai chi master who was so relaxed, so sensitive to the forces in and around him, that his whole body would sway gently under the impact of a fly landing on his shoulder. And there is the legend of another master on whose palm a bird had alighted; whenever the master sensed the bird tensing to take off, he would simply relax his hand and the bird would have nothing solid from which to take flight. However fantastic such legends may seem, it is the ability to be inwardly sensitive in the midst of action, to be relaxed and free enough to experience subtle variations in our sensations and feelings, which lies at the heart of our health and well-being. And it is through natural breathing that we can begin to experience this sensitivity and freedom.

PRACTICE

Be sure that you practice in a space where you won't be interrupted by people or phone calls. Though early morning is preferable, you can practice anytime during the day or early evening except for up to an hour after a meal. Wear as few clothes and as little jewelry as possible. Make sure that what clothes you do wear are loose, especially around the waist and pelvis. Do not practice outside if it is extremely cold or windy. When you practice, remember to be playful. Don't worry about results. As your breathing begins to reach into more parts of yourself, the results will come—usually when you least expect them.

Where appropriate, the practices in this book are divided into sections. Each new section builds on the previous section. Do not move on to a new section until you feel comfortable with the previous one.

1 Basic standing position

The following standing position will be used not just in this practice but in all other standing practices in this book. Don't worry if the position seems awkward at first. As you continue working with it, your body will begin to understand it through your inner sensation, and you will find yourself able to relax far more than you can in your normal standing postures. What's more, the posture will help root you to the earth and provide a stable foundation from which to experiment.

Stand quietly, with your knees slightly bent, your feet parallel (about shoulder width apart) and your arms at your side (Figure 10). Tilt your sacrum (the triangular bone that forms the back of the pelvis) very slightly forward, so that your coccyx (tail bone) is more or less pointed toward the ground and your lower back is flat (not arched). Let your knees bow slightly outward so that they are more or less over your feet. As you do this you will feel that both your perineum (the area between your anus and your sexual organs) and your groin are open. Let your shoulders and sternum relax downward and simultaneously feel that your head is being pulled upward from the crown, gently stretching the back of your neck.

2 Awakening attention

Once you are settled in the posture, sense as many parts of your body as you can simultaneously. Then let part of your attention focus on your feet. Sense the various points of your feet on the floor—the five toes, the pads under the big and little toes, the heel, and the entire outside edge of each foot. As you feel your feet relax, sense your weight sinking into and being supported by the earth. Once the sensation of sinking becomes clear, rock gently forward and back on your feet, from the ball of your foot to the heel and so on. Notice how various muscles in your feet, legs, and pelvis alternately tense and relax as your position changes in relation to the force of gravity. See if you can sense any adjustments in your back, your chest, your neck. Now shift your weight from side to side. See if you can simultaneously sense one leg becoming tense while the other relaxes. Let your attention take in as many sensations of these subtle

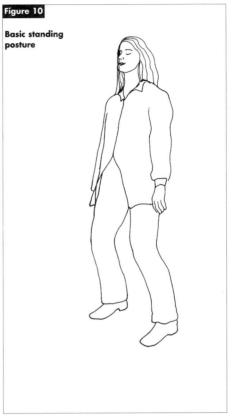

Figure 10

Basic standing posture

movements as possible. Work in this way for at least five minutes. Then stand quietly for a minute or two and sense any changes that have taken place in your overall sensation of yourself.

3 Basic sitting position

Now sit comfortably, either on a chair or cross-legged on a cushion on the floor, close your eyes, and sense yourself sitting there. Be sure that your spine is relaxed and straight and that you are not leaning against anything. Also make sure that the chair or cushion you sit on allows your hips to be higher than your knees. Rock forward and backward gently on your "sit bones" until you find a relative sense of ease and balance while sitting. Do not slump backward onto your tail bone (coccyx). This area is filled with nerves and is one of the body's key energy centers. Slumping back on this area will have a deleterious effect on both your awareness and your health. If your spine starts tightening up anytime during the practice, simply rock gently on your sit bones to help relax it.

4 Going deeper into sensation

Once you've found a comfortable yet erect sitting posture, let your thoughts and feelings begin to quiet down. One very effective way to support this "inner quieting" is by becoming interested in the overall sensation of your body. Start by allowing impressions of your weight and form to enter your awareness. Really let yourself sense your entire weight on the chair or floor. Once you can feel the weight clearly, include as much of the complete sensation of your skin as possible. When you can feel the tingling, the vibration, of your skin, then sense your overall form, the outer structure of your body, including any tensions in this structure. Sense yourself sitting there, letting your kinesthetic and organic awareness become increasingly alive. As your inner sensitivity increases, you will begin to experience your sensation as a kind of substance or energy through which you can begin to receive direct impressions of the atmosphere of your inner life.

5 Include your thoughts and feelings

Over time, as your sensation becomes more and more sensitive, you will begin to observe your thoughts and feelings as they start to take form— but before they absorb your complete attention. Let them come and go as they wish, but do not occupy yourself with them, analyze them, or judge them. As they come and go, simply include them in your awareness as part of the reality of the moment.

6 Include your breath

As you continue to work in this way, and as your inner attention becomes stronger and more stable, include your breath in your awareness. Follow your breath. Sense any movements or sensations associated with it. Let yourself really feel these movements of inhalation and exhalation, as well as their limitations and restrictions, in the context of the whole sensation of your body. Notice how your breathing influences your sensation of yourself. Don't try to change anything. Work in this way for 15 minutes or longer. You may want to try this practice morning and night for a week or two before continuing on.

AWAKENING ORGANIC SELF-AWARENESS

As we pointed out in the first chapter, our breath has an influence on all our major organs. Most of us, however, have little awareness of our inner organs. Few of us even know their locations in our body, and our doctors don't seem to have much interest in showing us. It wasn't until I reached my late forties that I even knew the difference between my small and large intestines, and where they were located. If you are one of those readers who is not familiar with the location of your organs, take a look at Figure 11. Study it carefully, seeing if you can sense the approximate location of the organs in your body.

As you undertake this work of organic self-awareness, it is important to recognize that though the internal organs and tissues are well supplied with nerves, the sensations in these areas are not as strong as sensations closer to the surface of the body, especially the skin. Pain in a particular organ, for example, is often "referred" by spinal nerve segments to other locations, so that it appears that the pain is coming from near the skin.

Internal organs

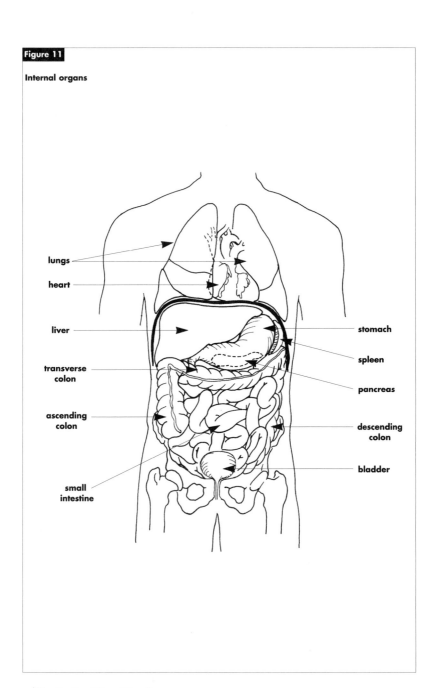

lungs

heart

liver

stomach

spleen

pancreas

transverse
colon

ascending
colon

descending
colon

bladder

small
intestine

For example, though it is well known that problems with the heart are often first felt in the arms, shoulders, and neck, it is not quite so well known that the uterus and pancreas refer pain to the lumbar region; the kidneys, to the groin area; and the diaphragm, to the shoulders.

PRACTICE

1 **Visualize and sense your internal organs**

Sit in the basic sitting posture. Visualize and sense the location of each of your internal organs. As you attempt to sense your organs, use your hands when possible to rub or probe around them. Start with the easiest organ to sense: the small intestine (in the area of the navel). Then move on to your liver (on the right side of the rib cage), and to your stomach, pancreas, and spleen (all more or less on the left side of the rib cage). Then sense your colon, your large intestine. (The colon extends from the end of the small intestine near the right hip bone up the right side of the abdomen and loops around to the liver area behind the ribs on the right side of the trunk. It then crosses the front of the body somewhere between the sternum and the navel, loops around behind the ribs on the left side of the trunk, and drops down toward the left hip. Near the left hip it angles toward the center of the body and turns into the rectum.) Now bring your attention to your heart (more or less in the center of your chest), your lungs (on each side of the heart), and your kidneys (protected by the lowest ribs on each side of the midback). As you touch these areas gently with your hands, feel the muscles and tissues around the organs begin to relax. Spend at least a couple of minutes sensing each area.

2 Sense the outer movements of your breath

Next, put your hands over the lower part of your chest, with the bottom edge of each hand touching the bottom of the lowest ribs, and the tips of the middle fingers touching each other at the bottom of the sternum. This is the area where the front of the diaphragm is attached to the ribs. The center portion of the diaphragm is actually higher, approximately at the level of the nipples. Observe your breathing. See if you can sense which way the diaphragm moves as you inhale and exhale. Don't use force. Don't try to change anything. Simply watch and sense.

Next, put your hands over your navel. Can you sense any movement in your belly as you inhale and exhale? Now put your hands over the lower ribs on the front of your body. What movements can you discern on the inhalation? On the exhalation? Next, put your hands on your lower ribs on both sides of your body. What happens as you inhale? As you exhale? Now put your hands on each side of your lower back in the kidney area (just opposite your navel, around the second or third lumbar vertebra). Again, see if you can sense any movement as you inhale and exhale. Next, put your hands on your upper chest. Notice what happens as you breathe in and out. Be sure to include in your awareness any tensions and restrictions in your breathing. Give yourself at least two or three minutes in each position.

3 Go deeper into your sensation

Now, try the same practice again. But this time, let your attention go deeper into your sensation. As you sense the movements of your breathing, let yourself experience how your internal organs are influenced. Put your hands over the middle of your chest as you did earlier. Can you sense your diaphragm putting pressure on any of your organs as you inhale? Which ones? What happens when you exhale? Now put you hands over your navel. What happens in the area of your small intestine as you inhale and exhale? Next, put your hands over the lower ribs in the front of the body. Sense what happens in the area of your liver on the right side and your stomach and pancreas on the left.

Continue on in this way following the same sequence as you did in the previous practice.

4 Include your emotions

Try the practice again. But this time include any sensations of warmth, coolness, dryness, or dampness in and around your organs. At the same time, take note of any emotions that may be present. Be careful not to dwell on them, analyze them, or judge them. Just include them in the field of your perception as you go on sensing yourself. It is as though you are taking inner snapshots of yourself through the wide-angle lens of your sensation—your inner organic awareness of yourself.

This is a foundation practice—one that you can and should return to daily. Later, once you become more proficient at taking inner snapshots of yourselves in quiet circumstances, you may find yourself quite spontaneously taking these inner snapshots when you are with other people. But be patient. Learning how to observe, through sensation, the interrelationships of your breath, tissues, organs, and emotions is a crucial step in both self-healing and wholeness. It will not only help make you more aware of the unconscious attitudes that create stress in your life, but it will also begin to free you from these attitudes. Most of the practices discussed in future chapters will build on this practice of organic self-awareness, and will expand on the ideas put forward in this chapter.

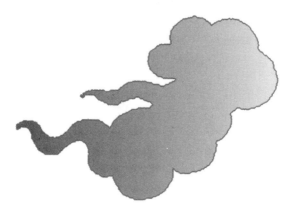

THE TAOIST VISION OF ENERGY AND BREATH

For the Taoist, the conscious cultivation
of breath offers a powerful way
not only to extract energies from the
outside world but also to regulate
the energetic pathways of our inner world,
helping to bring our body, mind,
and emotions into harmonious balance.

In many traditional cultures, breath is envisioned as a direct manifestation of spirit. It is the subtle energy of the spirit that "enlivens" us, and we receive this subtle energy by breathing it in or having it breathed into us from above. Terms such as *prana* (India), *pneuma* (Greece), *lung* (Tibet), *num* (the Bush people of Kalahari), *ruach* (Hebrew), *ney-atoneyah* (Lakota Sioux), *baraka* (Islam), and *chi* (China) are just a few of the many names of this higher life force upon which we are said to depend. And it is through our own authentic breath that we can consciously connect with this life force.

Though Western science rejects any notion of a subtle energy or life force that animates us, it does, like many of the traditions, believe that we live in a universe of energy and energy transformations, and that we depend on these energies to think, to feel, to move, and so on. For the Western scientist, these energies—which include mechanical, chemical, electrical, radiant, and nuclear—are defined in relation to the "work" they can do. This work must, however, be measurable through the techniques of hard science, especially through instrumentation designed for that purpose. By definition, anything that cannot thus be measured does not exist. Of course, other researchers, including some in "softer" sciences such as psychology and psychiatry, have over the years posited the existence of subtle energies with names such as bioplasma, bioelectricity, biocosmic energy, and so on. And they, too, have often defined these energies in relation to the work they can do—especially in relation to our own minds and bodies. They have not, however, fared well in a society geared to the marriage of science, technol-ogy, government, the medical establishment, and the drug industry.

One of the most famous of these energy researchers is Wilhelm Reich. On the basis of much experimental evidence and personal verification by many people, Reich maintained the existence of a powerful life force energy which he called *orgone* energy. He began to show people how to use this energy to help prevent and fight various life-threatening diseases, including cancer. Since he viewed his work as experimental, he did not charge his patients. Yet the U.S. federal government moved against him, and in May 1956, in response to his refusal to obey FDA injunctions, the government sentenced Reich to prison, where he died of a heart attack in November 1957. While he was in prison, the FDA raided his institute and burned his books and other writings.[22]

THE REMARKABLE ENERGY OF CHI

It is only today, after the documented success of certain forms of "alternative medicine," including meditation and Chinese healing arts such as acupuncture and chi kung healing (*chi kung* means *energy cultivation*), that a few open-minded pioneers in the Western medical community have begun to accept the possibility that there may be subtle forms of energy, such as chi (also written *qi*), that Western science has not yet learned to measure. The 1994 PBS television series and companion book by television journalist Bill Moyers, *Healing and the Mind*—which documented some of the latest breakthroughs in mind/body research by psychologists, neurologists, and immunologists—devotes a section to "the mystery of chi." Moyers draws no definite conclusions from his experiences in hospitals and elsewhere in China, but he does admit to seeing "remarkable and puzzling things."[23]

Since long before the birth of Christ, Taoist and chi kung masters have been experimenting with remarkable and puzzling things—with the subtle energies and functions of the body and psyche. Through their own personal practices with breathing, posture, movement, sensory attention, visualization, sound, and meditation, they have discovered how to beneficially influence not only our thinking and feeling, but also the various internal systems of the body, including the enzymes, hormones, blood cells, and other vital substances and energies that lay at their foundation. The effectiveness of many of these practices has been verified over the past two decades by chemical and biophysical research done by scientists in collaboration with respected chi kung masters in some of the top universities and laboratories in China—research that has shown the remarkable influence of chi on everything from crystals to the human immune system.

Chi and Negative Ions

Taoists and chi kung masters maintain that, in principle, we can all learn how to use chi to promote health and well-being. They believe, for example, that the process of breathing not only draws in the oxygen needed by the body to transform food into chemical energy through the flame of internal combustion, but that it also provides an entrance-way and support for the various other energies that animate our being. From the modern Taoist's perspective, for example, the discovery by modern science that the earth's atmosphere is filled with electrical charges called *ions* is highly significant. Some Taoists have even gone so far as to identify negative ions with chi. Ions are either positively or negatively charged atoms or parts of molecules. Negative ions, which are tiny packets of almost pure electrical energy, are formed naturally by interactions of the sun's energy with our atmosphere, as well as by cosmic particles, lightning, storms, winds, the evaporation and movement of water, and low levels of radioactivity coming from the earth. Thousands of scientific studies have shown that ions, especially negatively charged ones—those which carry an extra electron—are extremely important to our health. In commenting on research that was done in France in 1966, for example, one author writes that "in the lungs the presence of negative ions favors the passage of oxygen through the air cell membranes so that this oxygen is more efficiently absorbed by the blood. At the same time, the removal of carbon dioxide is also made easier."[24] And according to Robert Ornstein, Ph.D., and David Sobel, M.D., "Negative ions have been shown to increase brain serotonin, a neurotransmitter associated with more relaxed moods."[25]

Studies have also shown that negative ions are constantly being depleted as a result of pollution, air conditioning, closed spaces, concrete buildings, artificially generated electrical fields, deforestation, and so on.[26] These studies, of course, come as no surprise to Taoist masters, who prefer to undertake practices for health and spiritual growth in the midst of nature—near mountains, lakes, rivers, forests, and so on—where negative ions are most abundant. The importance of negative ions has become increasingly recognized in science and industry, and ion generators have become widely available for home and office, as well as for automobiles. Many Japanese businesses now have air-conditioning systems with ion generators. They are even being used in space capsules to help astronauts overcome tiredness and various psychological maladies. My Taoist teacher, Mantak Chia, frequently refers to the importance of negative ions, and to the use of special breathing practices to absorb them into the body.

Taoists use many special breathing techniques, including swallowing the breath directly into the digestive tract,[27] to absorb and transform energy in the atmosphere, including negative ions, not only for meditation and spiritual awareness, but also for self-healing and longevity. For the Taoist, the conscious cultivation of breath offers a powerful way not only to extract energies from the outside world but also to regulate the energetic pathways of our inner world, helping to bring our body, mind, and emotions into harmonious balance. Taoists believe that it is this balance, the beginning of real wholeness, that lies at the heart of health and well-being.

THE "THREE TREASURES"

As a result of thousands of years of experimentation and observation, Taoists maintain that human life depends on the unobstructed movement and transformation of three main forces, which Mantak Chia calls "earth force," "cosmic force" (the higher energy of self, of nature), and "universal force" (the energy of the heavens, of the stars). In the human organism, these forces manifest as three different substances or energies—the "three treasures": *ching,* sexual essence; *chi,* vitality or life force; and *shen,* spirit. We receive these energies from several main sources: from our parents (heredity), from the food we eat, and from the air we breathe. Though we are generally not aware of it, we also receive them directly from the earth, nature, and the stars through the soles of our feet, our skin, our palms, the crown of our head, and other energy centers of the body. According to Mantak Chia, numerous Taoist practices are designed to teach how to better attune to, absorb, and digest these energies.[28]

Inner Alchemy

Taoist practices are also directed to a kind of inner alchemy—the transformation of sexual essence into vitality, and vitality into spirit—both for health and for spiritual evolution. This transformation takes place in the three main energy centers of the body, called "tan tiens," or "elixir fields"—located in the lower abdomen, the solar plexus, and the brain. It is in these centers that the real alchemy of the human organism takes place. The energies circulate from these centers through various energy pathways, called meridians, that bring energy to all parts of the organism (Figure 12). In Western terms, the tan tiens and meridians are roughly analogous to electrical generating and transforming stations that create electricity from various raw materials of different density and efficiency— such as coal, oil, and natural gas—and deliver this power through a complex network of wires to our homes and thus to our appliances.

"ORIGINAL CHI"

One of the most crucial forms of energy for our overall health and well-being is the energy we receive through heredity—from the sexual union of our parents, of yin (female essence) and yang (male essence). This is called "original chi."[29] A major part of our original chi is our sexual essence, or ching, so we will not discuss ching separately. According to Mantak Chia, our original chi is stored mainly in the lower tan tien, in the center of a triangle formed by the navel, the point on the back

Figure 12

Meridian pathways of the body

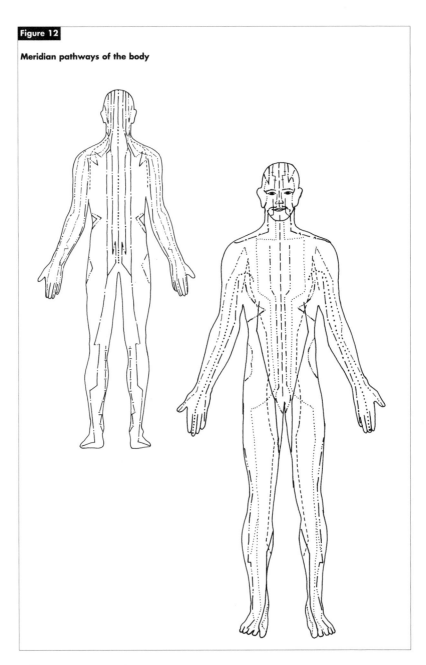

midway between the kidneys, and the sexual center (in the area of the pubic bone). The exact location of this center, which varies depending on a person's weight and structure, is about one to two inches below the navel and approximately one third of the way in (Figure 13). The lower tan tien is the basic storage battery of the body, providing the core energy needed for the combustion and transformation of the energies we receive from food, air, and so on.

From the Taoist perspective, an abundance of energy in the lower tan tien makes it easier to assimilate all the other forms of energy available to us. This energy center, like all the others in the body, is a kind of magnet that can attract outside energy with a corresponding vibration. The Taoists would say, "where there is more, more is given." They would also say, without much overstatement, that our health and well-being begins with keeping a certain reserve of energy in the appropriate energy centers of our organism, especially in the lower tan tien, the area of our sexual essence or vitality. When we sense energy in this area, we generally feel balanced and centered. When our energy is blocked in this area, or when we have insufficient reserves, we may feel a general physical weakness and imbalance. We may also catch ourselves behaving in judgmental or critical ways toward ourselves and others. Our energy can be blocked or lost in a variety of ways, including excessive negativity, tension, stress, daydreaming, talking, and sexual activity, as well as through gossip, criticism, worry, and so on. Although some of the lost energy is replenished automatically through eating and breathing, our original chi gradually dissipates as we grow older.

We can, however, learn to intentionally "conserve" our energy and to "recharge" our battery—to keep our lower tan tien open and filled with energy—through mindfulness (awareness) practices with the help of special breathing practices. Two of the most basic of these breathing practices are *normal abdominal breathing* and *Taoist abdominal breathing*. Normal abdominal breathing, in which the belly, rib cage, and lower back expand on the inhalation and contract on the exhalation, has a variety of benefits, including an automatic massage of the inner organs

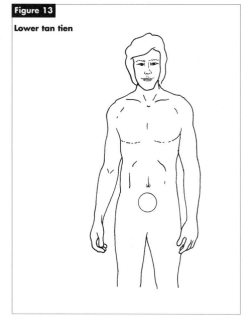

Figure 13

Lower tan tien

and an increased flow of chi around these organs. "It also helps to promote the flow of blood, lymph, and hormones, and ... reduces the work of the heart."[30] This form of breathing is similar to the soft, natural breathing of a baby or young child. Lao Tzu makes reference to it in the *Tao Te Ching* when he says: "Focus your vital breath until it is supremely soft, can you be like a baby?"[31] The other basic form of breathing, called Taoist abdominal breathing or "reverse" breathing (since the belly, sides of the rib cage, and lower back go inward on inhalation and outward on exhalation) compresses and packs the energy in the lower tan tien and the surrounding organs. It also aids in the circulation of this energy through the meridians. We will explore reverse breathing in Appendix 1.[32]

PRACTICE

As we saw in Chapter 2, one of the keys to health and healing is the work with self-sensing—the development of inner attention and awareness. Without this work with our inner attention and the eventual ability to control it, the breathing practices described in this book will have little impact. In discussing the importance of attention, an acknowledged master of chi kung and Chinese medicine writes: "By attention we mean both the experience of consciousness and the activity of the brain that lies behind it. Regulating attention allows the practitioner to bring his/her Qi into a comfortable condition. Finding this state of comfortableness and ease is the key to successfully apply Qi Gong to eliminate disease, strengthen the body, prolong life, and promote intelligence."[33] What is crucial in these breathing practices is thus to undertake them with full clarity, effortlessly and comfortably, that is, without strain, without any effort to achieve some result that you think you *should* have. Also give yourself plenty of resting time after each practice, so that you can sense its influence on you.

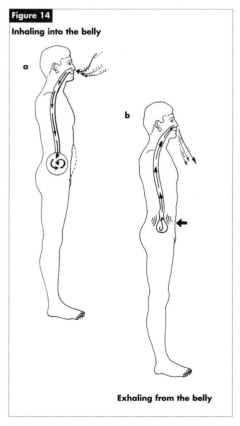

Figure 14

Inhaling into the belly

Exhaling from the belly

1 **Opening your belly**

Sit or stand quietly. Observe how you breathe for several minutes, then put your hands over your navel. As you inhale, sense that you're breathing directly from your nose through a long narrow tube into a balloon behind your navel. As the balloon expands, so does your abdominal area. As you breathe out, the balloon contracts and you have the sensation that the air is squeezed slowly back up through the tube and out through your nose (Figure 14). Obviously, the air that you inhale does not go into the abdomen; it goes into the lungs. But the "sensation" of a movement going from the nose into the abdomen relaxes your abdominal muscles and tissues and helps the diaphragm move lower into the abdomen and massage your inner organs. Be sure that your shoulders and chest remain relaxed during this exercise. *Do not use effort.* Simply visualize and sense the movement of the balloon in your belly. Simultaneously sense the downward and upward movement of the diaphragm as you inhale and exhale.

2 Sensing your diaphragm

To get an even clearer sense of the movement of your diaphragm, lie on your back with your knees bent, your feet slightly apart and flat on the floor, and your arms at your side (Figure 15). As you inhale into your belly, let the balloon expand as much as possible. At the end of the inhalation, hold your breath, making sure that no air can escape through your nose or mouth. Then, without breathing, gradually flatten your belly and gently shift the balloon of air up into your chest. Simultaneously, sense your diaphragm moving upward. Now flatten your chest and shift the balloon back down into your belly. See if you can feel your diaphragm moving downward at the same time. Move the

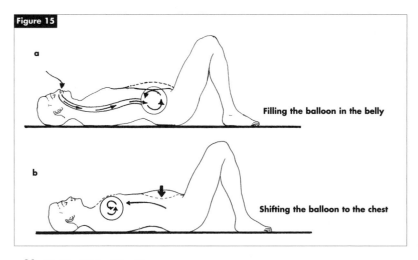

Figure 15

a

Filling the balloon in the belly

b

Shifting the balloon to the chest

balloon back and forth several times in a pumplike motion. Rest for a couple of minutes and observe any changes in your breathing. Try the exercise two or three more times.

3 Opening your rib cage

Continuing to lie on your back, put your hands on the sides of your rib cage over your lower ribs and feel the expansion of the balloon into both sides of the rib cage as you inhale. As you exhale, the ribs return to their normal position. By breathing in this way, you are helping the diaphragm to move even deeper into your abdomen, since the bottom of the diaphragm is attached to the lower ribs. To get an even better sense of the movement of your rib cage, lie on your right side with your head resting on your right arm and your left palm resting gently on the lower left side of your rib cage (Figure 16). As you breathe, feel that you are breathing directly into and out of the left side of your rib cage. Work in this way for 15 or 20 breaths, and then lie again on your back with your feet flat on the floor. Sense your breathing for several breaths—notice if there is a difference between the left and right sides of your rib cage. Now lie on your left side with your head resting on your left arm and your right palm resting on the lower right side of your rib cage. Breathe into the right side of your rib cage for 15 or 20 breaths. Again lie flat on your back with your knees bent, breathe gently into both sides of your rib cage, and sense any changes in your breathing.

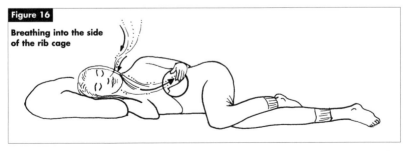

Figure 16

Breathing into the side of the rib cage

4 Opening the "door of life"

Sit or stand comfortably again, putting your hands on each side of your spine on your lower back (tips of the fingers actually touching the spine), directly across from your navel. The Taoists call this area, between the second and third lumbar vertebrae, the "mingmen," or the "door of life," since it is the point between the two kidneys where our sexual essence is stored. It is very important from the standpoint of our well-being to keep this area warm, relaxed, and comfortable. As you inhale, sense the balloon filling and pushing your lower back outward (Figure 17). As you exhale, your lower back returns to its original position. Breathe in this way for two or three minutes. To get the feeling of the movement of your lower back in the process of breathing, try squatting. Squatting is useful not only for opening up the lower back, but also for your overall health. As you squat, let your arms relax forward, and sense your lower back as you breathe (Figure 18). This posture automatically releases the lower back muscles, as well as the lower part of the diaphragm, which is attached to the lumbar spine. It also helps cleanse and energize the kidneys. If you have trouble squatting, you can stand and bend over with your upper body supported by your hands on

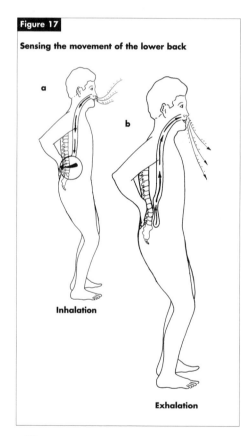

Figure 17

Sensing the movement of the lower back

a

b

Inhalation

Exhalation

your knees. Once you feel the sensation of your lower back expanding and contracting in this way, return to a normal sitting or standing position, and let the "organic memory" of what you just experienced help you sense the same process in this position.

5 Opening the belly, rib cage and lower back simultaneously

Next, either sitting or standing, try to experience all three areas at the same time. Sense the entire space bounded by your navel, your pubic bone, and your lower back. As you inhale, sense the balloon expanding forward, backward, and to the sides more or less simultaneously. As you exhale, sense the balloon contracting. There should be no feeling of effort or tension. Simply sense the balloon filling and emptying. Be sure to sense your diaphragm moving downward as you inhale, and upward as you exhale. After a few minutes, forget the balloon and simply feel the warmth in your abdomen, a kind of ball of energy, expanding and contracting. As you breathe naturally in this way, begin to sense that even though air is not going into the abdominal cavity, "something" is going there. From the Taoist perspective, this something is both blood and chi. By breathing in this way you begin to energize your lower tan tien. You can try this practice several times a day.

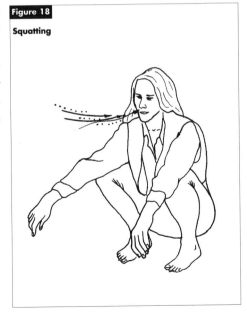

Figure 18

Squatting

"ACQUIRED CHI"

The energy that we acquire through food, water, and air is called "acquired chi." This is the energy that we receive from the outside world that we need to function on a daily basis. The main center for the storage and transformation of this energy is the middle tan tien, located in the area of the solar plexus, the center of our emotional life. For the Taoist, the quality of this energy depends in part on the quality of the food we eat and the air we breathe. The Taoist is therefore not only concerned about right diet, but also about right breathing.

As we have seen, proper breathing has many benefits besides the more efficient consumption of oxygen. The practice of abdominal breathing, for instance, has a powerful influence on the digestion of food by increasing gastrointestinal peristalsis, blood flow, and food absorption. It can also help open the tissues around the solar plexus and promote the flow of energy through the channels in this area. According to Mantak Chia, when this area is blocked or energetically weak, we may feel panic or worry, a lack of freedom in our behavior, or an inability to take risks of any kind. We may also feel that we are unloved or incapable of love, or that people are constantly judging us.

Abdominal breathing—especially when it is slow, deep, and long—combined with certain mindfulness practices directed to specific energy centers, can also help us receive the energies of the earth, nature, and the heavens. This form of breathing turns on the parasympathetic nervous system, which calms our brain and body. This allows our inner attention to clearly sense vibrations, impressions, and movements of energies in and around us that are ordinarily invisible to us. It is the sensing of these vibrations, as well as of the centers that can receive them, that allows these energies to be absorbed into our organism.

PRACTICE

1 Opening your solar plexus

Sit or stand quietly and watch your breath for several minutes. Now put your hands over your abdomen and feel the energy ball behind your navel expanding as you inhale and contracting as you exhale. Allow your awareness to go deep inside the tissues in your abdomen. After several breaths, let the energy ball spread, during the inhalation, from your navel area up into your solar plexus (located slightly higher than midway between your navel and the bottom of your sternum). As you exhale, sense the solar plexus and navel areas contracting. As you begin to relax into your inner sensation, your breath will gradually slow down by itself. Put your hands over your solar plexus, and bend over slightly from your waist. See how your breath responds. Repeat this several times. Then stop the bending and bring all your attention to the solar plexus area. Watch how it expands and contracts with each inhalation and exhalation. Work in this way for several minutes.

2 Releasing deep tensions

When you begin to feel your solar plexus becoming more sensitive and open, sense the air going from your nose through your solar plexus and into your lower tan tien (Figure 19). Envision the air as a long thread of silk connecting the whole front of your body from your nose down to your abdomen. As you exhale, breathe out through your mouth. Make sure your mouth is mostly closed, and that your exhalation is slow, quiet, and steady. Allow all the air in your lungs to be exhaled fully before inhaling again. As you exhale, sense that all the tension in your abdomen, solar plexus, and chest is going out through your breath. Breathe quietly in this way for five or 10 minutes. Pay special attention to the area around your solar plexus. Feel it become continually softer, as though something were melting. Then let go of any intention with your breath and simply take note of the various vibrations in and around your body. There's nothing to do but watch and sense. Work for at least 15 or 20 minutes in this way.

SHEN

Shen is generally translated as spirit or higher mind. It is also a substance or energy in the human body. Though shen can be either original or acquired, we will not differentiate it in this book. Sometimes called "celestial chi" because of its origin in the stars, this energy resides in the upper tan tien, the energy center located between the eyebrows in the area of the pituitary gland in the brain (Figure 20). This center controls the basic energy of the mind, the energy required both for clear thinking and for awareness. Shen is the light of lucidity, of consciousness, that shines through our eyes when we are awake. When this area is opened and energized we experience strong intuition and a sense of real purpose. When it is closed or weak, our attention is scattered and we feel distracted or indecisive. There are many stories of Taoist or Chinese doctors who will not treat someone in whom the light of shen is too weak. For without sufficient shen, without a certain level of "spirit," healing becomes impossible.

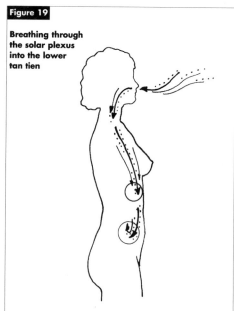

Figure 19

Breathing through the solar plexus into the lower tan tien

Shen Can Be Increased

A certain amount of shen is produced naturally in the organism. But given the various stresses of modern life, it is not always sufficient to keep us healthy, and it is seldom sufficient for psychological or spiritual transformation. But shen can be intentionally increased. One of the best ways to accomplish this is through conserving our basic life force, and supporting the transformation of this life force into the more subtle energy of awareness. This work depends in large part on being able to stay in touch with,

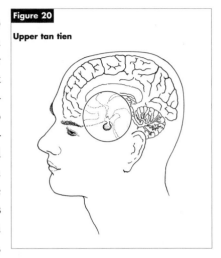

Figure 20

Upper tan tien

to sense, the area of the lower tan tien and learning how to keep this area open and active through awareness and proper breathing. Deep abdominal breathing not only helps move our life force into the higher centers where it can be transformed, but it also helps quiet the mind and calm the brain. This is important because as science has shown, "In the adult, the rate of brain activity, measured metabolically, is ten times that of any other tissue in the body at rest. In fact, the brain burns ten times as much oxygen and produces ten times as much carbon dioxide as the rest of the body."[34]

From both the scientific and Taoist perspectives, the brain's marathon activity influences the entire body, activating nerves, hormones, muscles, tissues, and organs. When the mind becomes quiet—when we can slow down or stop the unnecessary mental and emotional activities (such as daydreaming, criticism, self-pity, inner talking, and random associative thinking) that fill most of our day—the cells and tissues of the brain and body begin to rest and recuperate, spending less energy and storing more. This helps to increase the overall level of energy, of chi, in our organism. When chi reaches a certain level of intensity in the organism, and we are able to sense it through a quiet, ongoing awareness, transformation of more of this energy into the finer energy of shen happens naturally. This higher level of shen not only supports healing and well-being, but is also the foundation for psychospiritual growth.

PRACTICE

1 Opening your brain

Sit or stand quietly in the usual posture, allowing your mind to become quiet and your awareness to include as much of your entire organism and its functions as possible. After 10 or 15 minutes, put your attention just below your navel and sense the energy ball expanding and contracting as you inhale and exhale. Once you feel that you are in touch with this area, allow your attention also to include the upper tan tien between your eyebrows. Sense your eyes relaxing back into their sockets. Feel the entire area around your eyes relaxing. The actual experience feels like something hard softening, or like ice melting to become water. As this melting process takes place, observe any thoughts or feelings you may be having. Don't make an occupation out of these experiences. Let them go, and continue sensing.

2 Breathing into your brain

Once the area between your eyebrows feels soft and open, see if it is possible to inhale directly through this area into your brain, while simultaneously staying in touch with your deep abdominal breathing. See if you can feel a kind of subtle vibration, or movement, in this area. Don't believe the negative thoughts that may arise, thoughts that will undoubtedly tell you that it is impossible to breathe into your brain. Just try it. See for yourself. Work in this way for 10 minutes or so. When you are ready to finish, bring your attention (and your breath) back to your lower tan tien. Feel that any energy you have collected is somehow being stored there. Breathe quietly in this way for a couple of minutes before stopping.

In pondering the implications of the ideas and practices put forward in this chapter, do not worry about remembering the technical terms used here. What is important is to begin to sense that your own harmonious functioning depends on a variety of specific substances (or energies) coming from both inside and outside, as well as on the movement of these substances through your breath to the places in your body where they can be stored and transformed. As you work gently over a period of weeks with the ideas and practices described in this chapter, you will begin to feel a new sense of vitality and openness, especially in your belly, solar plexus, and face. Take note of this sensation. Let it begin to spread throughout your body. Return to it as often as you can.

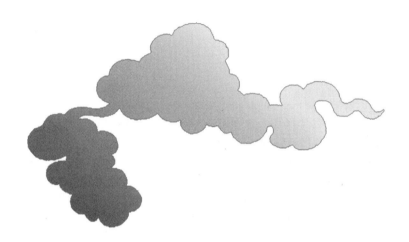

THE WHOLE-BODY BREATH 4

*... when we are able to breathe through
our whole body, sensing our verticality
from head to foot, we are aligning ourselves
with the natural flow of energy connecting
heaven and earth.*

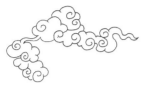

More than 2,000 years ago, the great Taoist philosopher Chuang Tzu said that "The True Man breathes with his heels; the mass of men breathe with their throats."[36] This ancient observation about breathing, which may be especially relevant today, lies at the heart of the Taoist approach to breath. For the Taoist, breathing, when it is natural, helps open us to the vast scales of heaven and earth—to the cosmic alchemy that takes place when the radiations of the sun interact with the substances of the earth to produce the energies of life. It is our breath, especially our "natural" breath, that enables us to absorb and transform these energies.

What is "natural" breathing? We began to answer this question in the first two chapters, when we reviewed the basic physiology of breathing and explored how to observe our breath in relation to our tissues and organs. We went deeper into the meaning of natural breathing in the third chapter, when we worked with the three primary energy centers of our body, especially the center in the area of the navel. In this chapter, we will expand the work we've begun to include the whole body in our breath. For it is only when our whole body breathes that we can gain the fullest access to our inner healing power—to the organic vitality that is our birthright.

A SIMPLE DEFINITION OF NATURAL BREATHING

One of the simplest, most practical definitions of natural breathing that I've found comes from the well-known psychiatrist Alexander Lowen, who studied with Wilhelm Reich. "Natural breathing—that is, the way a child or animal breathes—involves the whole body. Not every part is actively engaged, but every part is affected to a greater or lesser degree by respiratory waves that traverse the body. When we breathe in, the wave starts deep in the abdominal cavity and flows up to the head. When we breathe out, the wave moves from head to feet."[37]

From the point of view of this definition, most of us have little experience of natural breathing. In my healing work using Chi Nei Tsang (internal-organs chi massage), for example, many of the people I work on have, at the beginning of my treatments, little awareness of any movement in their abdominal cavity, lower ribs, and lower back. As I observe their breathing, or put my hands into their belly or on their chest, it is clear that the respiratory wave generally begins in the middle of the chest, or even higher, and seems to move only a short distance upward into the shoulders and neck. Some of these people have had abdominal surgery of some kind, and it is clear that even many years later they are still protecting themselves from feeling the pain of the surgery. Others are clearly protecting themselves from feeling painful emotions. Still others feel insecure about their sexuality. But what they all have in common is that they are unconsciously using their breathing to try to cut themselves off from feeling their physical and psychological discomforts and contradictions.

DISTINGUISHING THE OUTER AND INNER MOVEMENTS OF BREATH

To appreciate the true power of natural breathing, it is necessary to begin to distinguish two aspects of our breathing: the outer breath (the way in which our physiology operates to bring about physical respiration) and the inner breath (the subtle breath that circulates throughout our being). Whether we are working alone or being helped by someone with more experience, the key to natural breathing is through training our inner sensitivity, our inner awareness, to sense the various inner and outer movements of our breath as they take place. It is this sensitivity, and particularly its expansion into the unconscious parts of ourselves, that will enable us eventually to begin to sense the physical and emotional forces acting on our breath. It is only when we can sense these forces as they are—without any judgment or rationalization—

that our breath can begin to free itself from its restrictions and engage more of the whole of ourselves.

The Outer Movements of Breath

From what we've said so far, it is possible to discern at least two levels of movement in our respiratory apparatus during inhalation and exhalation. During inhalation, as the air travels downward through our nose and trachea, the diaphragm also moves downward to some degree into the abdomen to make room for the lungs to expand, while the belly expands outward to make room for the diaphragm. Thus the first movement that we can sense in natural breathing is the downward movement of the diaphragm and air. As the lungs begin to fill from the bottom, however, there is also a movement of the air upward—the kind of movement that occurs when we fill a glass or a bottle—which is reinforced by a movement of the chest outward and the sternum upward, creating more room in the middle and upper part of the lungs (Figure 21).

During exhalation, we can sense the air moving upward and out in concert with the diaphragm, which relaxes back into its original dome-like structure pushing upward. Simultaneously, we can sense the movement of the sternum downward and the ribs and belly inward, all of which bring about an overall relaxation of the whole body downward into the earth (Figure 22). Thus, whether we are inhaling or exhaling, we can sense two simultaneous movements going in opposite directions. Indeed, it is through the simultaneous sensing of these opposing movements of air and tissue that we begin to develop the kinesthetic awareness—the inner sensitivity—necessary to relax our tissues and discern the movement of energy in our organism.

The Inner Movements of Breath

From the Taoist perspective, the main issue in natural breathing is the movement of the actual "breath energy," the chi, in the organism. The movement of this energy is the result of the polarity between inhalation (yang, active, upward) and exhalation (yin, passive, downward),

Figure 21

Inhalation

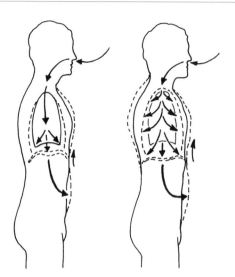

The diaphragm moves downward; the belly, chest, and lungs expand

Figure 22

Exhalation

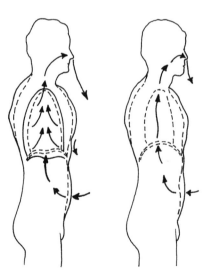

The diaphragm relaxes upward; the belly, chest, and lungs contract

between filling and emptying. The Taoists have observed that as we inhale, the breath energy moves upward to the head, and that as we exhale, the energy moves downward into the whole body. They have also observed that as we inhale, we can also draw the yin energy of the earth, a powerful healing energy, through our feet and upward into our body. As we exhale, we can direct any toxic or stagnant energies downward to our feet and out into the earth. The Taoists also maintain that during inhalation we can draw the yang energy of heaven directly into our body through the crown, the energy center on the very top of our head, and that during exhalation we can distribute this energy downward throughout our body (Figure 23).

THE POLARITY OF HEAVEN AND EARTH

Whether or not we believe in the energies of heaven and earth, we know that it is the polarity of positive and negative, of yang and yin, that creates electricity and makes energy move. We also know that there are various electromagnetic fields surrounding the earth, and that these fields are themselves manifestations of this fundamental polarity. An American firm that has produced negative ion generators for the space program points out, for example, that a natural electric field exists between the earth and the atmosphere, and that this field—which has a strength of several hundred volts per meter in an open space with unpolluted air—is usually positive in relation to the earth. The company also points out that experiments have shown that this field attracts negative ions from the upper atmosphere and produces an electric current in the body that stimulates living organisms in a beneficial way.[38]

The Taoists, of course, have spoken for thousands of years about the polarity of yang and yin, of up and down, of heaven and earth. As living organisms, we depend not only on chemical and electrical polarities within our bodies, but also on the electromagnetic polarity of the earth and atmosphere. As conductors within this electromagnetic field, our bodies manifest a potential difference in voltage between head (positive) and feet (negative) that increases in relation to the degree of our

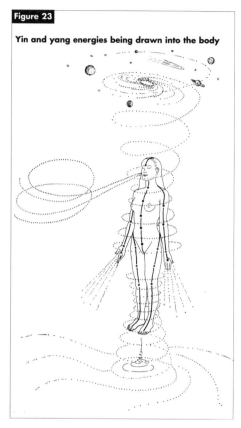

Figure 23

Yin and yang energies being drawn into the body

verticality. Other important factors include our location, the purity of the air, the climate, and so on. In a closed space with polluted air, for instance, the potential difference is virtually zero.

It is my belief that when we are able to breathe through our whole body, sensing our verticality from head to foot, we are aligning ourselves with the natural flow of energy connecting heaven and earth. This vertical flow may help to explain the great healing power of both tai chi and chi kung, especially when they are done, as recommended by Taoist masters, in fresh air and open spaces.

THE BENEFITS OF WHOLE-BODY BREATHING

In addition to bringing us into a more harmonious relationship with the energies of heaven and earth, whole-body breathing has a number of benefits at both the physiological and psychological levels. At the physiological level it not only increases our intake of oxygen and helps to promote efficiency in the entire breathing mechanism, but it also helps—through the internal massage it provides—to revitalize all the cells, tissues, and organs of the body, and to clear the body of any toxins. At the psychological level, whole-body breathing helps us relax enough to begin to experience ourselves from the inside out, to discover an inner attention that can take in more accurate, complete impressions of the whole of ourselves and our functioning. As this occurs—as our breath expands into hitherto unconscious parts of ourselves—our attitudes and emotions start to change and our self-image begins to release its stranglehold on our lives.

PRACTICE

Sit down and go through as many of the previous practices as time permits. When you finish these practices, let your awareness embrace the whole of your sensation. You will feel this sensation—including your skin, your tissues, your muscles, tendons, and ligaments, your organs, and your bones—as varying intensities of vibration, some denser, some finer. See how many levels of vibration you can discern.

1 **Sensing the outer movements of breath**

Now, within this field of sensation, begin to follow the movements involved in breathing. As you inhale, see if you can sense the downward movement of the air and your diaphragm. See if your belly expands as you inhale. If not, gently put your palms over your navel, and sense how the warmth from your palms begins to attract your breath and open your belly. As you exhale, see if you can sense the upward movement of the diaphragm and the inward movement of your belly. As you continue following these movements, notice how far they reach in your body. As you inhale, for example, see how far down the movement actually goes. Does the movement reach your pelvic floor? As you exhale, see how far up the movement goes. Does it reach your head? Don't try to "do" anything. Simply watch as your breath begins to take in more of your body. Work in this way for 10 minutes or so.

2 Sensing the inner movements of breath

As you continue to sense these upward and downward movements in the tissues of your body, include the movements of your "breath energy." As you inhale, see if you can sense some kind of energy, of vibration, rising upward into your head. As you exhale, see if you can sense this vibration moving downward through your whole body. Give yourself plenty of time. Using our inner attention to follow these movements is not something we are accustomed to doing. The key is to let go of any unnecessary tension and just keep "listening" to your sensation.

3 Making contact with your head and feet

Next, sense your feet resting firmly on the floor. Allow them to relax, as though they were spreading out over and even down into the floor. As they relax, you may begin to feel a vibration at the point in your foot called "bubbling springs" (the Kidney 1 acupuncture point at the upper part of the middle of your foot, as shown in Figure 24). Allow that vibration to spread into your whole foot, and even upward into your leg. Then, for a minute or two, massage the crown point at the top of your head with your index and middle fingers (Figure 25). Rest and sense the point opening. You may feel this opening as a subtle vibration, a melting, a prickly sensation, or a kind of numbness. In any event, keep your attention there until you experience a sensation of some kind.

4 Sensing your whole body breathing

As you keep your attention on your feet and crown you will begin to sense your whole body involved in breathing. As you inhale, you may feel as though you are drawing the bubbling sensation in your feet all the way up through the tissues and organs of your body to join with the breath energy moving to the top of your head. As you exhale, you may sense the inner energy of your breath spreading downward through your entire body toward your feet. When this happens, just enjoy this sensation of the breath energy moving upward and downward in your

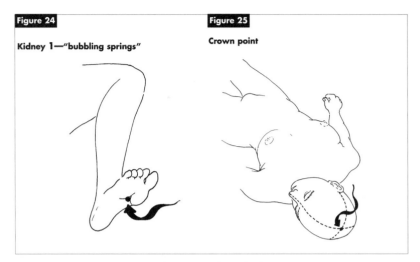

Figure 24

Kidney 1—"bubbling springs"

Figure 25

Crown point

body. Observe any areas where your breath does not seem to penetrate or move. Work for at least 10 minutes in this way, simply observing the rising and falling of energy, of sensation, through your body. If you don't feel these movements yet, don't worry. This can take time. Just go on to the next practice.

5 Lengthening your spine

Stand again in the basic standing posture, with your knees slightly bent and your feet parallel, about shoulder width apart. Let your shoulders relax and your arms simply hang at your sides. Put your attention on the bubbling springs point on both feet and on the crown point. Feel the vibration in both areas. Allow your inhalation to rise from your feet and go all the way up to and out through the top of your head. As it moves up through the top of your spine and your head you may, especially during your first few breaths, sense your spine being lengthened and your head being pulled upward so that it rests more lightly on your spine. Allow your exhalation to start from the top of your head and go down through your feet into the earth. Be sure to stay in touch with your spine as you exhale; see if you can maintain its length. Feel as though your breath is simultaneously raising you upward and rooting

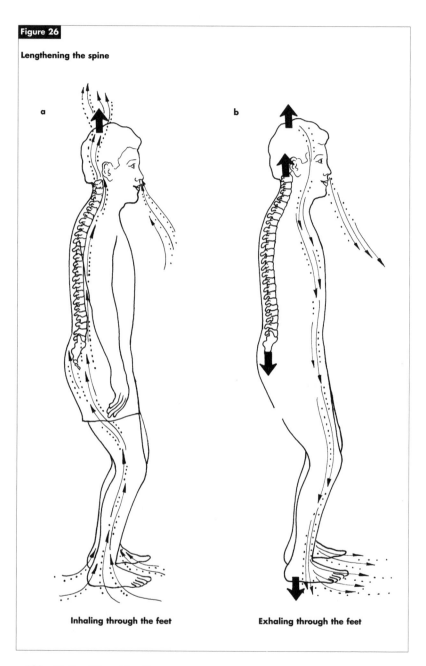

Figure 26

Lengthening the spine

a

b

Inhaling through the feet

Exhaling through the feet

you downward (Figure 26). Don't think about the irrationality of this experience—just let it happen.

6 Connecting heaven and earth

Once you've been able to sense these movements, try the following exercise using the same basic standing position. As you inhale, slowly rise up on your toes, and simultaneously raise your arms up in front of you. Your arms should arrive straight over your head (palms facing forward) at the same time that you have reached your full extension (Figure 27). As you exhale, slowly lower your arms and feet until you are in the original standing position. Try this many times. Sense the upward and downward movement of energy. Sense your whole body breathing. Experience how your breath is putting you in touch with your own verticality—connecting heaven and earth both inside and outside your body. Once you've felt this, walk around for a few minutes and see how long you can maintain this sensation.

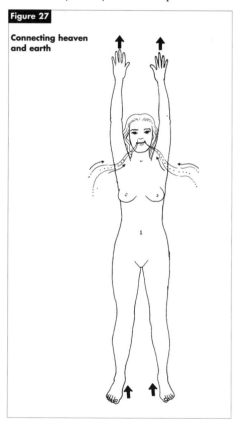

Figure 27

Connecting heaven and earth

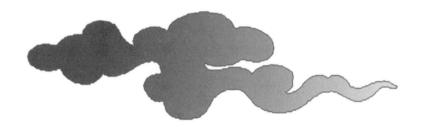

THE SPACIOUS 5 BREATH

... each breath we take is filled
not only with the nutrients and energies
we need for life, but also with the expansive,
open quality of space. It is this quality
of spaciousness, if we allow it to enter us,
that can help us open to deeper levels
of our own being and to our own
inner powers of healing.

Thirty spokes together make a wheel for a cart.
It is the empty space in the center
of the wheel which enables it to be used.
Mold clay into a vessel;
it is the emptiness within
that creates the usefulness of the vessel.
Cut out doors and windows in a house;
it is the empty space inside
that creates the usefulness of the house.
Thus, what we have may be something substantial,
But its usefulness lies in the unoccupied, empty space.
The substance of your body is enlivened
by maintaining the part of you that is unoccupied.[39]

Lao Tzu

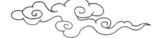

To experience the natural healing power of breath is to experience its inherent "spaciousness." Our breath can not only move upward and downward to help us experience our own verticality, but it can also move inward and outward to expand and connect our inner spaces with the space of the so-called outer world. In the same way that our experience of external space allows us to differentiate and relate to each other and the various objects and processes of the outer world, our experience of the internal spaces, the "chambers" of our bodies and psyches, allows us to differentiate the various functions and energies of our organism and keep them in dynamic harmony. As Chuang Tzu states:

"All things that have consciousness depend upon breath. But if they do not get their fill of breath, it is not the fault of Heaven. Heaven opens up the passages and supplies them day and night without stop. But man on the contrary blocks up the holes. The cavity of the body is a many-storied vault; the mind has its heavenly wanderings. But if the chambers are not large and roomy, then the wives and sisters will fall to quarreling. If the mind does not have its heavenly wanderings, then the six apertures of sensation will defeat each other."[40]

Clearly, for Chuang Tzu and the Taoists, the various chambers or stories of the human organism—especially the abdomen, chest, and head—need to be experienced as "large and roomy" if our various functions and energies are to work in full harmony. Without some sense of spaciousness in our organs and tissues, we are unable to feel space in the other aspects of our lives. It is just this feeling that there is no space in our lives, that there is no room to expand our experience of ourselves, that lies at the root of much of our stress and dis-ease. It is one of the main reasons we so cherish trips to the countryside or ocean, where we find not only expansive vistas of land and sky, but also profound, inexhaustible silence. Though these spacious experiences of our eyes and ears help open up our psychological structure, including our feelings and mind, the sense of spaciousness and silence quickly disappears when we return to our ordinary circumstances.

The Tibetan Buddhists also put great emphasis on the importance of space to our well-being, making clear that the "feeling of lack of space, whether on a personal, psychological level or an interpersonal, socio-logical level, has led to experience of confusion, conflict, imbalance, and general negativity within modern society.... But if we can begin to open our perspective and discover new dimensions of space within our immediate experiences, the anxiety and frustration which results from our sense of limitation will automatically be lessened; and we can increase our ability to relate sensitively and effectively to ourselves, to others, and to our environment."[41]

LEVELS OF SENSATION

The discovery of "new dimensions of space within our immediate expe-riences" lies at the foundation of health and inner growth. Because our most immediate experience is the sensation of our own body, it is here that we can most effectively begin this discovery. The sensation of the body can be experienced at many different levels, and it is just this organic experience of various levels, of various densities of sensation, that begins to give us a taste of internal spaciousness. These levels include the sensation of superficial aches and pains; the compact sensation of the weight and form of the body; the more subtle sensation of temperature, movement, and touch; the tingling sensation of the totality of the skin; the living, breathing sensation of the inner structure of the fascia, the muscles, the organs, the fluids, and the bones; and the integrative, vibratory sensation of the body's energy centers and pathways.

But there is one more level of sensation that we are given as our birthright. This is the all-encompassing sensation of openness that lies at the heart of being. As our sensation begins to open up, as we sense a broader frequency of vibration in our experience of ourselves (a vibration that *includes* instead of excluding), we come into touch with the sensation of the energy of life itself—before it is conditioned by the rigid mental, emotional, and physical forms of the society in which we live, and, even more importantly, by our own self-image. As we learn more and more about how to allow this direct sensation of life into our experience of ourselves, we feel a growing spaciousness, a sense of wonder in which the restrictions of our self-image can begin to dissolve. It is the organic experience of this essential spaciousness that embraces the various polarities and contradictions of our lives, the various manifestations of yin and yang, and allows them to exist side by side in our being without reaction. This inner, organic embrace, this sensory acceptance of everything that we are, frees not only our body but also our mind and feelings, bringing us a new sense of vitality and wholeness.

THE THREE BREATHING SPACES

To experience this inner, organic embrace, however, requires that we begin to open up the various chambers of our being, allowing them to return to their original "large and roomy" condition. The most direct way to begin this process is to learn how to experience the essential spaciousness of our breath and to guide this spaciousness consciously into ourselves—into what Ilse Middendorf calls our "three breathing spaces." These spaces are the lower breathing space, from the navel downward; the middle space from the navel to the diaphragm; and the upper space from the diaphragm up through the head (Figure 28). By learning how to breathe into and experience these spaces, we begin to open to ourselves in new ways. We learn how to relax all unnecessary tension and to find dynamic relaxation, the ideal balance between tension and relaxation, in our own tissues—in the various boundaries of these spaces. And this work, in itself, can bring about many important changes both in our perception of ourselves and in our health.

The idea of the three breathing spaces coincides from an anatomical standpoint almost exactly with the concept of the "triple burner," or "triple warmer," in Chinese medicine. The triple burner is one of the basic systems of the body, a system with a name and a function but no specific form. It consists of an upper, middle, and lower energetic space, each of which contains within it various organs. From the standpoint of Chinese medicine, the triple burner integrates, harmonizes, and regulates the metabolic and physiologic processes of the primary organ networks. It is associated with the overall movement of chi and is also responsible for communication among the various organs of the body. It is my experience that consciously bringing the breath into

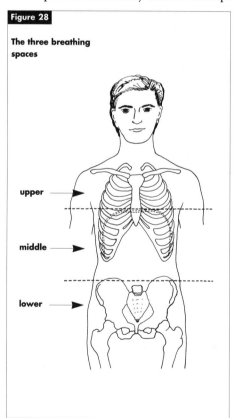

Figure 28

The three breathing spaces

upper

middle

lower

each breathing space, into each burner, and sensing the spacious movement of the breath up and down through the spaces and the organs within these spaces, has a powerful balancing effect on my physical and psychological energies. If I work with this practice before I go to bed at night, it calms me and helps me sleep better; if I work with it during the day, it brings me a sense of greater relaxed vitality.

This work with the breathing spaces of the body is extremely powerful. In writing about the results of her approach to the breath through working with the various breathing spaces of the body, for example, Middendorf points out that "Through practicing and working on the breath we constantly create and experience new breathing spaces. This enables the body to free itself from its dullness and lack of liveliness, so that it feels easy and light through the continuing breathing movement and filled with new power, it feels good and more capable. This dynamic way of breathing can lead to great achievement and success in every expression of life. With its healing power it also reaches symptoms, states of exhaustion, depressions. An increasing ability to breathe will prevent these states from occurring anymore."[42]

Whatever theoretical framework we may choose for understanding our work with breath, each breath we take is filled not only with the nutrients and energies we need for life, but also with the expansive, open quality of space. It is this quality of spaciousness, if we allow it to enter us, that can help us open to deeper levels of our own being and to our own inner powers of healing. In spite of its simplicity, however, spacious breathing is not an easy practice to learn. Years of conditioning and "ignor-ance" have left us not only with many bad breathing habits, but, perhaps even more importantly, with little kinesthetic awareness of our own physical structure, and with how this structure hinders or supports our breathing. Without this inner sensation of our structure, any attempt to impose a new way of breathing—whether yogic, Taoist, or any other form—on our organism can only lead to confusion, and, potentially, further problems.

PSYCHOLOGICAL OBSTACLES TO AUTHENTIC BREATHING

Once we begin to get in touch with the sensation of this structure, however, we will begin to become aware of the mental and emotional forces acting on our breath, on our own particular rhythms of inhalation and exhalation. This is a crucial aspect of any serious work with breathing, since it will show us the psychological obstacles to discovering our own authentic breath.

Our Inability to Exhale Fully

According to Magda Proskauer, a psychiatrist and pioneer in breath therapy, one of the main obstacles "to discovering one's genuine breathing pattern" is the inability that many of us have to exhale fully. Whereas inhalation requires a certain amount of tension, exhalation requires letting go of this tension. Full inhalation without full exhalation is impossible. It is important, therefore, to see what stands in the way of full exhalation. For many of us, what stands in the way is often what is no longer necessary in our lives. Proskauer points out that "Our incapacity to exhale naturally seems to parallel the psychological condition in which we are often filled with old concepts and long-since-consumed ideas, which, just like the air in our lungs, are stale and no longer of any use."[43] She makes it clear that in order to exhale fully we need to learn how to let go "of our burdens, of our cross which we carry on our shoulders." By letting go of this unnecessary weight, we allow our shoulders and ribs to relax, to sink downward into their natural position instead of tensing upward. Full exhalation follows quite naturally.

Our Inability to Inhale Fully

Those of us who are unable to exhale fully in the normal circumstances of our lives are obviously unable to inhale fully as well. In full inhalation, which originates in the lower breathing space and moves gradually upward through the other spaces, one's abdomen, lower back, and rib cage must all expand. This, as we have seen in earlier chapters, helps the diaphragm, which is attached all around the bottom of the rib cage and anchored to the spine in the lumbar area, to achieve its full range of movement downward. For this to happen, the muscles and organs involved in breathing must be in a state of dynamic harmony, free from unnecessary tension. But this expansion is not just a physical phenomenon, it is also a psychological one. It depends on both the wish and the ability to engage fully with our lives, to take in new impressions of ourselves and the world.

Freedom To Embrace the Unknown

Full exhalation and inhalation are thus most possible when we are free enough to let go of the known and embrace the unknown. In full exhalation, we empty ourselves—not just of carbon dioxide, but also of old tensions, concepts, and feelings. In full inhalation, we renew ourselves—not just with new oxygen, but also with new impressions of everything in and around us. Both movements of our breath depend on the "unoccupied, empty space" that lies at the center of our being. It is the sensation of this inner space (and silence)—which we can sometimes experience in the natural pause between exhalation and inhalation—that is our path into the unknown. It is the sensation of this space that can enliven us and make us whole.

PRACTICE

To prepare for this practice, sit or stand quietly with your eyes open and experience the coming and going of your breath. Get in touch with the three tan tiens—just below the navel, in the solar plexus, and between the eyebrows. Sense the different qualities of vibration in these areas. As you breathe, sense your outer and inner breath—the various upward and downward movements of both tissue and energy. Clearly note any areas that seem to be tense or closed to your breath. Spend at least 10 minutes on this stage of the practice.

1 Opening your breathing spaces

During exhalation, use two or three fingers to press gently into your lower abdomen, between your pubic bone and your navel. During inhalation, gradually release the pressure. Sense how your abdomen responds to this pressure. Take several breaths this way. Now put your hands over your navel, and work in the same way—pressing as you exhale, and gradually releasing the pressure as you inhale. Notice how your lower breathing space begins to open.

Next, put your hands over your lower ribs on both sides of your trunk. As you exhale, gently press your ribs inward with your hands. As you inhale, gradually release the pressure from your hands and sense your ribs expanding outward. It is helpful to realize that the lower ribs, also called the "floating ribs," can expand quite freely since they are not attached to your sternum. In fact, the expansion of the floating ribs helps create more space for the lungs to expand at their widest point.

Now, apply light pressure to your solar plexus as you exhale. Again, watch for several minutes as your upper abdomen begins to relax and open. Next, as you exhale, press lightly on the bottom of your sternum. Taking several breaths in each position, gradually work your way up toward the top of the sternum. If you take your time and work gently, you will find your various breathing spaces beginning to become more elastic and spacious. Now try this same approach with any areas of your abdomen, rib cage (both on and between your ribs), shoulders, and so on that seem overly tight or constricted. Take your time. It is actually better to do this work for 15 or 20 minutes each day over a period of a week or so than to try to do it all in one session.

2 A simple technique for opening the three breathing spaces

There is another, simple technique that you can experiment with to help open the three breathing spaces. This technique, which I learned several years ago from Ilse Middendorf, involves pressing the appropriate finger pads of one hand against those of the other. To help open the lower space, press the pads of the little fingers and the pads of the ring fingers together firmly but without force. For the middle space, press the pads of the middle fingers together. For the upper space, press the pads of the thumbs and index fingers

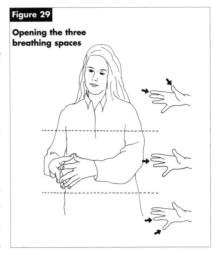

Figure 29

Opening the three breathing spaces

together. To help open all the spaces simultaneously, press the pads of all five fingers together (Figure 29). When you first begin this practice do not take more than take eight breaths while pressing your finger pads together.

3 Movement of spaciousness

Once you feel more of the whole of yourself involved in breathing, put most of your attention on the movement of air through your nose during inhalation. Take several long, slow breaths. Feel the empty, expansive, spacious quality of the air as it moves down through your trachea and into your lungs. But don't stop there. As you continue your inhalation, sense this spaciousness moving downward through all the tissues and organs of your abdomen and filling your entire lower breathing space. Allow this feeling of space to release any tensions and absorb any stagnant energies residing below your navel. As you exhale slowly, use your attention to direct these tensions and energies out with your breath. Then work in the same way with the middle breathing space (from the navel to the diaphragm) and with the upper breathing space (from the diaphragm to the top of the head), sensing the various tissues and organs inside these spaces. When you have worked with all three breathing spaces, stop working intentionally with the feeling of space and simply follow your breathing.

4 Sensing the breath of the spine

Now that you have some direct awareness of the three major breathing spaces, especially in relation to the front of the body, we're going to work with the inner space of the spine, the very core of our body, which connects the three breathing spaces in the back. In particular, we're going to sense the craniosacral rhythm of the cerebrospinal fluid as it pulses through the central canal of the spine, moving from the brain down to the sacrum. The cerebrospinal fluid—a clear fluid produced from red blood flowing through a rich supply of blood vessels deep within the brain—not only provides nutrients for the brain and spine, but also removes the toxic products of metabolism and functions as a shock absorber. The pressure of this fluid has an influence on nerve flow and affects the ability of the senses and brain to take in new impressions.

Lie down on your back with your legs stretched out and your arms at your side. Sense again the expansion and contraction of your breath as it moves through the three breathing spaces, the three burners. See if you can include your heartbeat in your sensation. After several minutes, put your fingers on your temples above your ears (you can rest your elbows on the ground) and sense the pulse of your heartbeat in your temples. Sense the way your head expands on inhalation and contracts on exhalation. You may also begin to feel the way your whole body takes part in this ongoing rhythm of expansion and contraction.

After two or three minutes working in this way, hold your breath intentionally after inhaling. See if you can sense an inner expansion and contraction radiating from the area of the head and spine. Make sure that you don't hold your breath for any longer than is comfortable. After taking several more spontaneous breaths, again hold your breath and touch the tip of your tongue to the center of the roof of your mouth. Later in the book we will go into the significance of this in completing the circuit of energy flow called the microcosmic orbit, but for now just see if you can sense the roof of your mouth expanding and contracting in rhythm with your head and spine. If so, what you are sensing is the pulsation of your cerebrospinal fluid. An entire cycle of expansion and contraction can take from five to eight seconds.

5 Sense your spine and breathing spaces at the same time

Now without losing touch with the "breathing" of your spine, include the three breathing spaces in your sensation of yourself. As you sense the pulsation of your spine, also sense the three breathing spaces as they empty and fill. As you exhale, the spaces contract from top to bottom. As you inhale, the spaces expand from bottom to top. *Don't force anything.* Just let yourself experience the process of natural breathing—a process in which the various spaces of your body all participate. Feel how with each breath the spaces are becoming "large and roomy." Let your awareness enter these spaces and enjoy the comfort of this natural process of expansion and contraction. After several minutes, get up and either sit cross-legged or on a chair. Continue to work with spacious breathing for several more minutes, noticing any changes brought about by your new posture.

6 The pause of spaciousness

Now simply follow your breathing. Notice the two pauses in your breathing cycle: one after inhalation and one after exhalation. Pay particular attention to the pause after exhalation. The great mystical traditions have spoken of this pause between exhalation and inhalation as a timeless moment—an infinite space—between yin and yang, nonaction and action, in which we can go beyond our self-image and experience our own unconditioned nature. See if you can at least sense this pause as an entranceway into yourself—into the healing spaciousness of your own deepest sensation of yourself. Don't try to force anything. Just watch and sense. Work like this for at least 10 minutes.

7 Spacious breathing under stress

It is relatively easy to have the sense of spaciousness when we are in quiet, undemanding circumstances. And it is important, especially at the beginning, to practice this kind of breathing in such circumstances. Eventually, however, you will want to begin to try spacious breathing, especially into your navel area, in the often stress-filled circumstances of your everyday life. For it is here that you will, with practice, have the largest impact on your overall well-being and health, and it is here that you will gain important new insights into your own nature. What's more, it is here that you will have an opportunity to discover a deep inner sensation of yourself that is somehow "separate" from the automatic reactions of your sympathetic nervous system (your "fight or flight" reflex), an overall sensation of yourself that will, if you can stay in touch with it, dissolve any unnecessary tension and bring about the appropriate degree of relaxation to meet the real demands of the moment.

To help prepare for working in such conditions, try the following practice. Stand with your weight balanced equally on both feet and your knees slightly bent. Sense the whole of yourself standing there, breathing. Let the sensation of yourself go deeper and deeper with each breath. Without losing this overall sensation of yourself, let your weight shift to your right foot. Bring your left foot up along the inner side of your right leg all the way up to your groin. Use your hands to help you position the heel of your foot in the area of your groin with your toes pointed upward if possible. Now raise your arms up from your sides (palms facing up) until your palms meet over your head (Figure 30). If this posture is too easy for you, if it does not arouse any stress, you might try closing your eyes and moving your arms up and down as you stand on one leg. If your health will not permit you to stand on one leg or to raise your arms above your head, then be inventive—find other ways to make the posture challenging for yourself.

Now, staying in this posture, let your chest and belly relax, and then begin to breathe into your lower abdomen. As you inhale, sense the spaciousness filling your lower abdomen; as you exhale, sense all your tensions going out with your breath. Breathe in this way for two or three minutes; then put your tongue to the roof of your mouth and see if you can also sense the pulsation of the cerebrospinal fluid. When you finish, slowly return your arms to your sides with your palms facing down and return to the original standing position with both feet on the ground. Sense your whole body breathing. Can you notice any differences between the left and right sides? Reverse your legs and repeat the entire process.

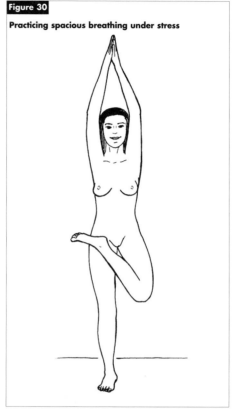

Figure 30

Practicing spacious breathing under stress

Because it is relatively difficult, this is an excellent exercise to prepare you to practice spacious breathing in the midst of tension and stress. The key is to learn how to relax inside this difficult posture. If you find that your belly and chest stay tense, put your attention on your face, ears, and tongue, and just let them relax. Because your face most directly reflects the tensions of your self-image, it is by learning how to relax your face that you can begin to relax the rest of your body. Try breathing directly into your entire face, especially in the area of the upper tan tien. Let space permeate your nose, eyes, ears, and so on. Then return to breathing in your lower abdomen.

If you begin to lose your balance at any time during this exercise, don't resist, don't try to compete with gravity. Whatever happens, stay in touch with the whole sensation of yourself, including your awkwardness (your body knows how to take care of itself without the help of your self-image). If you do fall, simply try again from the beginning. As you continue working in this way—not letting yourself react in the usual way to the difficulty of the posture or to your own awkwardness—you will begin to understand that this inner sensation of yourself is intimately related to a new, more inclusive level of awareness, a level of awareness that can transform your life.

8 Spacious breathing in the ordinary conditions of life

Once you are able to keep your belly, chest, and face relaxed during the previous practice, you are ready to try spacious breathing in the ordinary conditions of your life. Whatever you do, don't choose situations, especially at the beginning, that are so stressful that you will be doomed to failure. Start, rather, with ordinary situations—walking down the street, talking to a friend, and so on. Then, as you get a better feel of the practice in these conditions, you can move on to those that are more difficult. Eventually you will want to try spacious breathing when you are tense or emotional. Try it, for example, when you are in the middle of an argument with someone, or when you are lost in self-pity, anger, worry, impatience, and so on. If you are able to remember to practice in these more difficult conditions, you will experience first-hand how spacious breathing can help transform the stress and negativity that is bound up with your self-image into the energy you need for your own vitality and well-being.

As you undertake these practices, try them in a light, playful, and experimental way—from the standpoint of learning firsthand about yourself. As you continue this "playful" work with spacious breathing over many weeks and months, you will notice various tensions beginning to dissolve as if on their own. You will also notice your breath occupying more of each breathing space. These changes will make it possible for you to observe deep-rooted patterns of tension in the various postures and movements of your organism, patterns that inhibit the sensation of energy and movement and stand in the way of your becoming more available to the whole of yourself. You will also begin to sense that these patterns are related to, or even fueled by, various old attitudes and ideas, as well as chronic negative emotions, that create and maintain your self-image and leave little space for new experiences and perceptions. You may also observe that it is just these attitudes, ideas, and emotions that are the main obstacles to natural breathing and thus to your health and well-being.

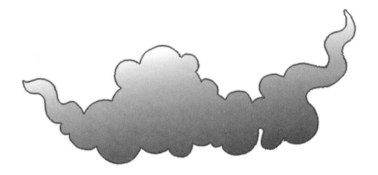

6 THE SMILING BREATH

*The "smiling breath" is for me a
fundamental practice of both self-awareness
and self-healing. The sensitive, relaxing energy field
that it produces helps me observe by contrast
the unhealthy tensions, attitudes,
and habits that undermine my health and vitality.
What's more, the practice helps to detoxify,
energize, and regulate the various organs
and tissues of my body, and thus helps
not only to strengthen my immune system but also
to transform the very way I sense and feel myself.*

Much has been written in recent years about the power of laughter to support the healing process. The story of how Norman Cousins, former editor of *The Saturday Review*, used laughter (and Vitamin C) to help recover from an incurable disease was first published in his book *Anatomy of an Illness* in 1979, and is widely known today.[45] In 1994, the California Pacific Medical Center in San Francisco, believing "that laughter is the best medicine," added a Humor in Medicine project to its Program in Medicine and Philosophy. According to the program's brochure, *Ways of the Healer,* "The physiological and psychological benefits of laughter have been well documented. This program addresses how to stimulate and apply healing laughter most effectively in a hospital setting."

THE CHEMISTRY OF A SMILE

Those of us who have experienced in our own lives how laughter can alter our emotions and support our well-being, may also have observed how a genuine smile from a friend—or even from a stranger on the street—is infectious and has the power to lift our spirits and release us, at least temporarily, from the restrictions of our stress and negativity. Such a smile can transform our physiological and emotional chemistry. It can bring new energy and a fresh perspective into our lives. It can help us "re-member" and accept who we really are. Yet, strangely, very little has been written about the chemistry of the smile and its relationship to healing.

The "Inner Smile"

Given the empirical evidence we have of the extraordinary power of a smile to bring about such changes, it is astonishing that so few of us intentionally smile on our own behalf. Taoist masters have long recognized the power of the smile to help transform our attitudes and energies. And this observation led them to begin to practice what Mantak Chia calls the "inner smile." In this practice we learn how to smile directly into our organs, tissues, and glands. "Taoist sages say that when you smile, your organs release a honey-like secretion which nourishes the whole body. When you are angry, fearful, or under stress, they produce a poisonous secretion which blocks up the energy channels, settling in the organs and causing loss of appetite, indigestion, increased blood pressure, faster heartbeat, insomnia, and negative emotions. Smiling into your organs also causes them to expand, become softer and moister and, therefore, more efficient."[46] One finds the inner smile used in a variety of Taoist meditations and other practices, including tai chi. One also finds versions of the inner smile in Buddhist literature (for example, in books by Thich Nhat Hanh), and artistic representations of it in the budding, self-aware smile of the Buddha or the Mona Lisa.

Voluntary Smiling Can Alter Our Emotional State

It doesn't take much observation or common sense to realize that intentionally "putting on a smile" can help change our emotional state. In his book *The Expression of Emotions in Man and Animals,* Charles Darwin observed that the free expression of an emotion by outward signs serves to intensify the emotion. Writing in the late nineteenth century, the great psychologist William James laid the foundation for a more complete understanding of this subject when he pointed out that emotions are dependent on "the feeling of a bodily state."[47] Change the bodily state or expression, and the emotions will change. More recently, Moshe Feldenkrais, one of the pioneers in physical rehabilitation and body awareness, has written that "all emotions are connected with excitations arising from the vegetative or autonomic nervous system or arising from the organs, muscles, etc. that it innervates. The arrival of such impulses to the higher centers of the central nervous system is sensed as emotion."[48] By changing the excitations coming from these parts of ourselves through a conscious change in our movements and postures we actually change our emotions, especially those emotions that support our self-image.

One could say, and quite reasonably, that there is a big difference between "spontaneous smiling" and "voluntarily smiling." In a recent scientific study on the effects of different kinds of smiles on regional brain activity, however, two researchers found that voluntary smiling actually changes regional brain activity in much the same way that spontaneous smiling does. In a discussion of their findings, the authors conclude: "While emotions are generally experienced as happening to the individual, our results suggest it may be possible for an individual to choose some of the physiological changes that occur during a spontaneous emotion—by simply making a facial expression."[49]

Relaxing Our Self-image and Regulating Our Organs

From the Taoist perspective, calling up a pleasant image that will bring about a smile—or even just putting a smile on one's face regardless of how sick or negative one may feel—has an almost immediate influence on the entire organism. It opens and relaxes one's face, which promotes openness and relaxation throughout the body. It also relaxes one's self-image and all the emotions and attitudes that support it. This deep relaxation helps to promote the appropriate movement of blood and energy in the organism for healing, and allows the brain and nervous system to better coordinate with and regulate the viscera.

Based on my own personal experiences, I believe that a sustained smile, especially a smile directed toward one's own organs and tissues, triggers the release of beneficial chemical substances from the remarkable pharmacopoeia that is the human brain—chemicals that can have an immediate healthful impact on the body. When I described the process of the inner smile to neuroscientist Candace Pert, and asked her if she believed that it could produce substances beneficial to the body, she replied "Absolutely." In going further into the question, she pointed out that peptides "modulate feeling," and she suggested that as we are "feeling," as we are "focussing on" an organ, as we are "paying attention to the autonomic circuitry" involved with it (curcuitry which is composed mainly of peptides), "we have the potential to regulate the organ."[50]

COMBINING THE INNER SMILE WITH SPACIOUS BREATHING

When the inner smile is combined with deep, spacious breathing to create what I call the "smiling breath," the effect can be even more powerful, since breathing can also influence the production of beneficial chemical substances in the organism. In the same conversation referenced above, Pert told me that one possible mechanism for the power that breathing has to alter our emotions and chemistry may be through the production of neuropeptides. She pointed out that the center that controls breathing is located at the fourth ventricle of the floor of the brain—the same location that also secretes many neuropeptides. And she suggested that by consciously altering our breath we may be able to influence which neuropeptides are released.

However one explains its power, the inward-directed smile is, experientially, like a beam of energy, of sensing and feeling, that guides the spacious breath deeper into the organism; and the spacious breath is like a carrier wave that transports the energy of the smile into all the organs. The "smiling breath" is for me a fundamental practice of both self-awareness and self-healing. The sensitive, relaxing energy field that it produces helps me observe by contrast the unhealthy tensions, attitudes, and habits that undermine my health and vitality. What's more, the practice helps to detoxify, energize, and regulate the various organs and tissues of my body, and thus helps not only to strengthen my immune system but also to transform the very way I sense and feel myself. The following smiling breath practice is based on my own experiments with combining certain elements of Mantak Chia's inner smile practice with what I call the spacious breath.

PRACTICE

To prepare for this practice, sit quietly for several minutes with your eyes closed. Sense your whole body simultaneously, including any tensions and emotions. Let these tensions and emotions begin to settle, like impurities in a glass of water. Don't stir them up by thinking about them. Include your breathing in your sensation of yourself. Then open up each of the three main breathing spaces through spacious breathing. Sense your whole body breathing.

1 Sensing and relaxing your eyes

Sense your eyes. Gently rotate, or spiral, them several times in each direction. Then stop and let them relax back into their sockets. As Mantak Chia points out, "The practice of the Inner Smile begins in the eyes. They are linked to the autonomic nervous system, which regulates the action of the organs and glands. The eyes are the first to receive emotional signals and cause the organs and glands to accelerate at times of stress or danger (the "fight or flight" reaction) and to slow down when a crisis has passed. Ideally, the eyes maintain a calm and balanced level of response. Therefore, by simply relaxing your eyes, you can relax your whole body and thus free your energy for the activity at hand."[51]

2 Let the sensation of relaxation turn into a smile

Once you feel that your eyes are relaxed, let the sensation of this relaxation spread through your whole face, even into your tongue and into the bones of your skull and jaw. Now visualize someone you care about smiling at you. Let their smile enter you, and smile back at them (Figure 31). Sense

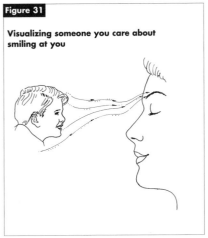

Figure 31

Visualizing someone you care about smiling at you

how your eyes and face relax even more. If you are unable to conjure up an image that makes you smile, then simply smile intentionally. Just turn up the corners of your mouth, raise your cheeks, and do the best you can. If you can maintain this effort for several minutes, you will soon find yourself smiling quite naturally.

3 Sense your face breathing through your smile

Now include your spacious breath in your awareness. Each time you inhale, sense the air entering not only through your nose, but also through your face and eyes. Sense your breath being touched by the smile on your face. Watch how the smile transforms your breathing. It's as though the smile makes your breath even more vibrant and expansive. As you continue to breathe in this way you may notice an increase in your saliva. This is a good sign. Don't swallow yet. Just keep breathing, collecting more and more saliva. Science has shown that saliva contains a wide variety of proteins, including hormones and other substances, that have digestive, antibacterial, mineral-building, and other health functions. The Taoists believe that in addition to these functions, the saliva—which they sometimes refer to as "the golden elixir"— can also readily absorb chi from our breath and help deliver this energy into the organism.[52] From the Taoist perspective, the increased production of saliva can, if utilized properly, be a great aid to our overall health.

4 Smile into your organs

Now you're going to guide your smiling breath into all your organs (Figure 32). Let your smile flow downward, like water, through your jaw and neck and into your thymus gland behind the upper half of your sternum. Sense the thymus gland opening and closing with each inhalation and exhalation. Then let the smiling breath go down into your heart. See if you can sense your heart relaxing as you smile and breathe into it. Then let the smiling breath expand into your lungs on each side of your heart. Can you sense your lungs expanding and contracting inside your chest? From your lungs, direct the smiling breath

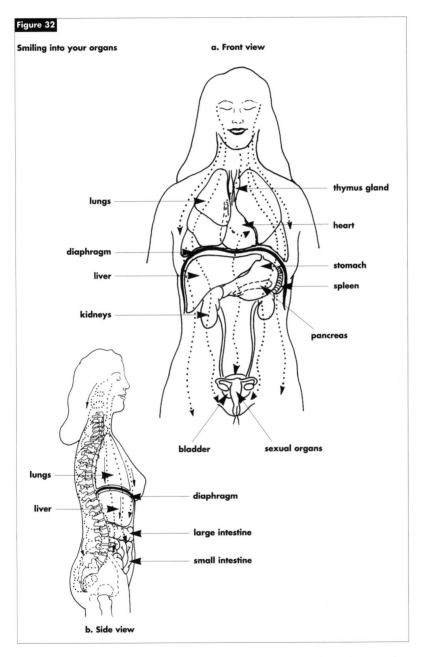

Figure 32

Smiling into your organs   a. Front view

- thymus gland
- lungs
- heart
- diaphragm
- stomach
- liver
- spleen
- kidneys
- pancreas
- bladder
- sexual organs

- lungs
- liver
- diaphragm
- large intestine
- small intestine

b. Side view

to your liver on the right side of your rib cage. Smile and breathe into this area. Sense the area around the liver expanding and contracting gently, and releasing any unnecessary tension. Now let the smiling breath include your pancreas and spleen on the left side of your rib cage, working in the same way that you did with the liver. Then include your kidneys, in the lower and middle back area. See if you can feel your back and kidneys expanding and contracting with each breath. Now let your smiling breath reach your bladder and sexual organs. As you breathe into this area, you may sense your whole lower abdomen opening and filling with energy.

5 **Swallow the saliva and follow your energy downward**

After completing this process, you will probably find your mouth secreting more saliva than usual. Let the saliva collect in your mouth. After collecting a sufficient amount, swish it around in your mouth several times and then swallow it at the very same moment that you straighten your neck slightly by tucking in your chin. As you swallow the saliva, you will sense a kind of warmth, a feeling of energy, leading your smiling breath downward into your body. Sense this sensation flowing slowly downward through your neck into your esophagus, stomach, small and large intestines, and rectum—right down to your anus. Sense your smiling breath going through your entire digestive tract.

6 **Bring the smiling breath into your brain and spine**

Return to spacious breathing and check again to be sure you have a smile on your face. Sense your eyes and let them relax back into their sockets. Feel as though your smiling breath is entering your body through your eyes and face and going back toward your pituitary gland, hypothalamus, and other parts of your brain (Figure 33). As you breathe in this way, you may feel that you are somehow becoming more conscious of your brain and its processes. Let your smiling breath go all the way to the back of your brain, in the area of the cerebellum. Sense that your whole head is beginning to expand and contract with your breath. Then let your smiling breath flow slowly down your spine, vertebra by vertebra, to your tailbone.

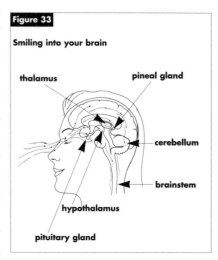

Figure 33

Smiling into your brain

thalamus

pineal gland

cerebellum

brainstem

hypothalamus

pituitary gland

7 Collect and absorb the energy

Now, as you inhale, sense your abdomen expanding with the spaciousness of your smiling breath. Sense the warmth and energy in your abdomen. As you exhale, do so gently through your mouth. Keep most of your attention in your abdomen and allow the comfortable, spacious sensation that you have there to spread simultaneously into all your organs, tissues, and bones. Once you feel that your awareness of this process is strong enough, you can add one more element to this practice. As you exhale, you can not only sense the "smiling energy" being absorbed into your organs, but you can also sense any inner tensions or toxins going out with the exhalation. As you gain proficiency in this practice, you will discover that it has enormous power to energize you and support your well-being.

As you practice the smiling breath, it is important to remember that its purpose is not to turn you into a smiling automaton. Its purpose is twofold: first, to help you make conscious contact with your own physical and emotional being, and second, to help free up your energies from unnecessary tension and negativity, from any area in yourself where you are "stuck." As you undertake the practice, check frequently to be sure that you still have a smile on your face. Eventually, after several months of practice, you will be able to bring about some of the same results with just the slightest sensation of an inner smile. This will allow you to practice the smiling breath in the midst of the stresses and conflicts of your daily life.

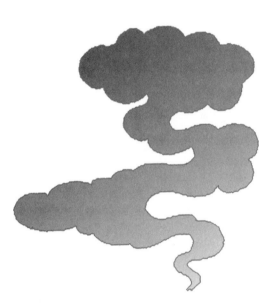

7
CIRCULATING THE VITAL BREATH

*Where our breath goes, our attention can also go.
By learning how to breathe naturally—
that is, by learning how to breathe vitality
into every corner of our being—we not only
promote the expansion of our inner consciousness,
but we also stimulate the healthful,
harmonious movement of substances
and energies throughout our bodies.*

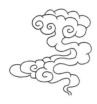

Our health and well-being depend on the constant and harmonious movement of energy, of chi, throughout the whole of our organism—energy that Taoists believe comes not only from food and air, but also from nature and the stars. From the flow of blood and lymph, to the movement of the cerebrospinal fluid, to the flow of nerve impulses and the firing of synapses, to the continual release of hormones and enzymes, to the reception of perceptions and impressions through our inner and outer senses, a healthy organism is one in which the movement of substances and energies continues unimpeded as needed through the various tissues, organs, nerves, vessels, and channels of the body. A blood clot, for example, can result in a stroke and instant death. Congested lymph nodes can promote disease. A "pinched" nerve can result in the loss of movement or sensation. Unnecessary tension in our muscles and tendons wastes energy, reduces our organic sensitivity, and contributes to the build-up of toxins in our organism.

THE NEED FOR NEW IMPRESSIONS

What's more, if we begin to observe our psychological life, we see that it functions analogously with and in close relationship to our physical life. Rigid beliefs and attitudes, as well as excessive emotionality (whether positive or negative), can be as dangerous to our well-being as plaque-filled arteries, since they can dramatically alter or impede the overall flow of our energy and diminish our inner and outer sense of spaciousness. Such psychological states can, if they become chronic, throw our entire system out of balance. Our experiences of ourselves can become so narrow that we lose any real sense of our own wholeness. Some great teachers, such as Buddha and Gurdjieff, use words such as *attachment* and *identification* to describe the process by which we lose touch with ourselves. When we continually "identify" ourselves with, or get swallowed up by, a particular image, idea, attitude, sensation, or emotional state, our awareness of ourselves, others, and our environment becomes extremely narrow. In addition, the circulation of energy in ourselves becomes disharmonious, and parts of ourselves do not receive the physical and psychological nutrition they need for health and well-being. What's more, such identification reduces what Gurdjieff calls the "food of impressions" through which "nature transmits to us ... the energy by which we live and move and have our being."[53] The flow of life, of energy, of impressions slows down, and we soon find ourselves exhausted—or even ill.

In my own history, it has become clear to me that my well-being has suffered most when my life seemed stale and devoid of movement, when it lacked new impressions of myself and the world, when it lacked organic satisfaction and meaning, or when there were simply too many impressions of one kind. At these times, I was caught, frozen, in a self-made prison of physical, emotional, and mental attitudes that excluded anything new from entering. It is clear not only experientially, but also scientifically, that the nervous system and brain need the constant but balanced stimulation of new impressions for both health and growth. As researchers Robert Ornstein and David Sobel point out: "The brain apparently has a need for a certain amount of stimulation and information to maintain its organization. When there is either too much or too little, instability results and disease may follow."[54]

Nourishing the Brain and the Immune System

For most of us, the stimulation the brain needs arises mainly through our contact with the outside world, through social interaction, entertainment, study, travel, job challenges, and so on, and this stimulation helps, *if it is not overly stressful,* to keep the organism in balance and to nourish the immune system. Every sensory impression we take in influences us. Even the taste and smell of food can have a nourishing affect on the immune system. A recent Duke University study showed, for example, that enhancing foods with powdered flavors and odors gave elderly participants, all of whom had taste and smell deficits, significantly higher levels of B and T cells. These lymphocytes, which mature in the bone marrow, thymus gland, and other areas, are "the strike force that, most often, rids bodies of infection and disease."[55]

New Flavors of Ourselves

The nourishment of the brain and the immune system through appropriate stimulation and information, however, is not dependent only on the perception of outer events. It can also occur through the perception of inner events, such as our ever-changing thoughts, feelings, and sensations. Self-observation and self-sensing enable us to experience new "flavors" of ourselves. They allow us to take in and metabolize direct impressions of our inner functions, attitudes, and energies. These impressions not only bring us a new sense of vitality, but they also begin to break down the confines of our self-image and give us a truer, more comprehensive sense of ourselves.

As we have seen, however, learning how to take in new impressions through self-sensing requires great inner relaxation. It also requires the ability to breathe into more of the whole of ourselves. Where our breath goes, our attention can also go. By learning how to breathe naturally—that is, by learning how to breathe vitality into every corner of our being—we not only promote the expansion of our inner consciousness, but we also stimulate the healthful, harmonious movement of substances and energies throughout our bodies.

MOVING OUR VITAL BREATH
THROUGH THE MICROCOSMIC ORBIT

From the Taoist perspective, the natural movement of energy, of chi, in our organism is, in fact, the movement of our "vital breath." This movement is governed by the law of yin and yang, which corresponds to the law of polarity, to the negative and positive charges of electricity and magnetism, and takes place through a complex network of energy pathways associated with the various sense organs, internal organs, and energy centers of the body. Energy flows from areas of greater "electrical" potential to areas of lesser potential. Illness and disease occur when this flow becomes blocked or unbalanced in some way. The channels can be opened or brought back into balance through a variety of means, including acupuncture, herbs, massage, meditation, special movements and postures, and, of course, work with breathing.

Based on their own observations and discoveries, Taoist masters and Chinese physicians believe that there are some 60 major energy channels, or meridians, in the human body. While some of these channels, called "primary channels," guide the vital breath (our life force) to the various organs and glands of the body, others, called "psychic channels," serve as special energy reservoirs connecting and feeding the primary channels. To understand the power of natural breathing from the Taoist perspective, it is necessary to explore the two main psychic channels: the governor channel and the functional channel. For it is these two channels that connect the main energy centers in our bodies. And it is these centers that absorb and transform our energy as it moves through them, and then supply the appropriate energy to the primary channels for distribution to the entire organism.

The Governor and Functional Channels

The *governor channel,* a yang channel, starts at the perineum (between the anus and sexual organs), moves back to the tip of the coccyx and up through the outside of the sacrum, and then rises up through the spinal column. When it reaches the skull, it continues to run upward along the surface of the brain up to the crown. From here, it descends through the middle of the face (about an inch and one-half below the surface of the skin) and ends at the palate at the top of the mouth. The *functional channel,* a yin channel, also starts at the perineum, rises up under the pubic bone and continues up the center line of the front of the body through the navel, solar plexus, and heart at depths of one to one and one-half inches until it reaches the tip of the tongue. In general, energy moves up the governor channel and down the functional channel, although it can move in the opposite direction as well. The energy circuit is completed between the two channels most efficiently when the tip of the tongue is touched to the roof of the mouth. This circuit is called "the microcosmic orbit," or "wheel of life," (Figure 34) and is the basis of Taoist alchemy for both health and spiritual growth.[56]

The Direct Sensation of Energy

Though our lives depend on the continuous circulation of energy through these two channels, the quantity, quality, and movement of this energy is often insufficient for the high level of health and vitality that is our birthright. From the Taoist perspective it is only through the direct sensation of this energy that we can correct this situation. Mantak Chia makes this clear when he writes that "Knowledge of the energy flow in our bodies makes it easy to understand why the Microcosmic Orbit must be kept actively open to accommodate and enhance the movement of Chi. When we do not know how to conserve, recycle, and transform our internal force through this pathway, our energy consumption becomes as inefficient as a car that only gets five miles per gallon. By practicing the Microcosmic Orbit meditation, we can get in touch with our Chi flow and locate blockages or weak spots in its path so we can correct them. This will help us use our life-force more efficiently and achieve better internal 'mileage.'"[57]

Most of us, if we are able to be honest with ourselves, have to admit that we have little direct sensation not only of our life force but even of the major parts of our body—our belly, chest, head, and back. When we do have a sensation of these areas it is generally through some kind of discomfort, such as back pain, indigestion, headaches, and so on—signals that our energy is stuck in some way or not moving properly. Through working with the microcosmic orbit, however, we begin to sense these areas more frequently in the course of our lives, along with any tensions that may be developing. What's more, our awareness gradually expands inward and we begin to have more-direct impressions of

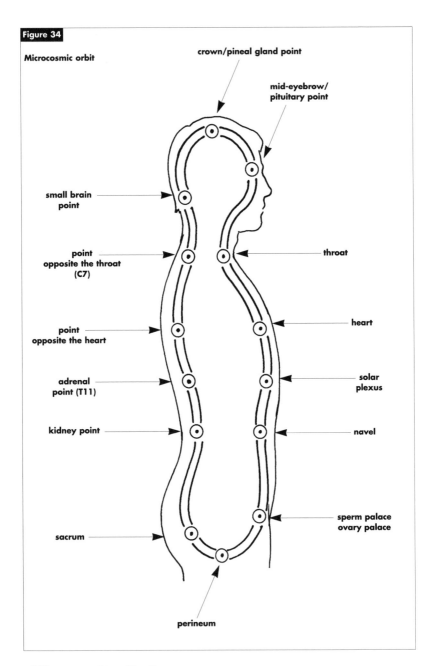

Figure 34

Microcosmic orbit

crown/pineal gland point

mid-eyebrow/
pituitary point

small brain
point

point
opposite the throat
(C7)

throat

point
opposite the heart

heart

adrenal
point (T11)

solar
plexus

kidney point

navel

sperm palace
ovary palace

sacrum

perineum

our bodies from the inside out, in relation to the movements and blockages of our life force. As we learn how to experience it directly through our sensation, the microcosmic orbit manifests itself as an ever-present pathway into the inner spaces and energy centers of our being. It is through impressions of the circulation of our internal energies within the framework of these spaces and centers that a real transformation can take place in our body and psyche—a transformation that can support both our health and our inner development.

PRACTICE

As I describe it here, the circulation of the vital breath is based on the microcosmic orbit meditation (as taught to me by Master Mantak Chia), a meditation that until recently was passed down only from teacher to student, and only after a student had demonstrated a high degree of commitment and perseverance. *Do not undertake this practice until you have worked through all the preceding material in this book and have begun to awaken your inner sensation in relation to the whole of your body.*

When working with the circulation of the vital breath, it is important to be in a relaxed, receptive state—a state in which you are open to receiving new impressions of yourself. As you will see from Appendix 2, each of the energy centers of the microcosmic orbit has specific psychological attributes associated with it, depending on whether the center is open or closed. Eventually, through self-sensing, you will begin to receive direct impressions of the condition of each center—and thus of your emotional and psychological state.

To prepare for this practice, begin by working for 10 minutes or so with the smiling breath, breathing into your various internal organs. Then spend several minutes breathing gently into your abdomen.

Sense your belly expanding as you inhale and contracting as you exhale. As this sensation becomes clearer, give up any effort and just allow your breath to rise and fall spontaneously. Take your time. See if you can sense that you are being "breathed" from deep within your abdomen.

As you undertake this practice, don't dwell too long on any one center, especially the centers of the heart, point opposite the heart, and head. Before the microcosmic orbit is completely open, keeping your attention too long on any one center can disrupt the flow of energy in your body. Don't focus on the heart, point opposite the heart, and head centers for more than 20 to 30 seconds each. For the other centers, one to two minutes each should be sufficient.

1 Awakening the energy of your perineum

Put your attention on the energy center in your perineum, between your sexual organs and your anus. Sense this area as clearly as you can. Once you have some sensation of this center, especially of its vibration, breathe into the area with a long, slow inhalation (Figure 35). Feel how the center seems to expand with your breath. As you exhale, let go of any tension in the area, any grasping or trying. Repeat this process until you can sense the energy in your perineum coming to life.

2 Awakening the centers of the governor channel

Now, allow your attention to begin to move up the governor channel to your coccyx and sacrum. (You may even find your attention going there quite spontaneously.) If you have trouble sensing this or any other area, use your fingers to probe it. Then work with your breath in the same way you did with your perineum. Once you begin to sense the area opening, move on, one by one, to the kidney point, opposite the navel; thoracic 11, opposite your solar plexus; the point between the shoulder blades, opposite the heart; cervical 7, which is the large vertebra at the base of the neck; the jade pillow, which is at the base of the skull; the crown point, at the very top of your head; and the mid-eyebrow point, which we worked with in earlier chapters. Don't try to force the sensation. Just allow each point to begin to open by itself as a result of the energy of your breath touching it. You don't need to go through all the points of the governor channel in one sitting. You can spread them out in 10 or 15 minute sessions over several days. If you do spread them out, however, start again with the perineum with each new session and quickly review the points you've already sensed.

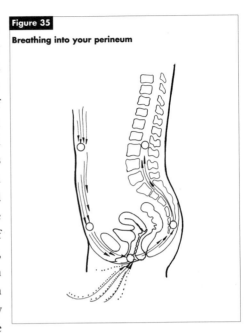

Figure 35

Breathing into your perineum

3 Awakening the centers of the functional channel

When you finally reach the mid-eyebrow point, touch the tip of your tongue lightly to the roof of your mouth just behind your upper teeth, and keep it there for the duration of the practice. (A good location is about where your tongue would go naturally when you say the letters "le" of the word *let*.) Now let your attention begin to go down the functional channel through your mouth and tongue to your throat center. Again, breathe into and out of this center until you begin to sense a vibration of opening. Then let your attention go in turn to your heart center, about one and one-half inches up from the bottom of your sternum; your solar plexus, about three quarters of the way up between your navel and the bottom of your sternum; your navel; your sexual center, in the area of the pubic bone; and finally back to the perineum. Take your time with this work. Impatience will only get in the way. What is important is to begin to actually feel the vibratory sensation of each center.

4 Circulating the vital breath

Once you can locate and sense the various centers, the next step is to begin to experience your breath energy as it circulates through them. This is not an easy practice. The Taoist classics make clear that sensing the microcosmic orbit in its fullness can take many years. It is important to remember that most of us have little experience working with our attention and energy in this way. For most of us, the energy centers are jammed up with tension and are barely discernible to our awareness. As a result, the process of opening the centers can on occasion be uncomfortable. As you continue to practice gently, however, you will begin to experience a new sense of movement in yourself, and much more direct contact with your energetic presence.

On the surface, the practice is quite simple. As you inhale, sense the breath energy moving up the governor channel from the perineum through the various centers. As you exhale, sense the energy moving down the functional channel from your mid-eyebrow point through the various centers and back again to your perineum. Be sure that the tip of your tongue stays in contact with the roof of your mouth. You can also occasionally try reversing the process—breathing up the functional channel, and down the governor channel. This will help clear the channels of any tensions or toxins. Don't worry if you can't sense some kind of movement through all the centers. Simply observe what takes place—where you can sense yourself and where you can't. Over time, the channels and centers will begin to open more fully, and you will receive new, direct impressions of your inner energies as they move more efficiently through your organism.

In the Taoist tradition the microcosmic orbit is also sometimes referred to as the "the small orbit." The Taoists also work with the "macrocosmic orbit," or "large orbit," in which the vital energy is moved not only through the governor and functional channels, but also through channels in the legs and arms. And there are still further practices that involve other energy pathways deep in the interior of the body as well. Unfortunately, many people begin working with these "higher" practices before they have laid the proper foundation for such work. This can lead not only to confusion, but also to physical or psychological harm.

HEALING AND BALANCE

Breathing through the microcosmic orbit is itself an advanced healing and meditation practice that is the basis of most of these other practices. It can have powerful effects not only at the level of our physical health, but also at the psychological and spiritual levels. Chi kung masters through the centuries have said that when you can experience energy flowing through the microcosmic orbit, hundreds of illnesses can be avoided or cured. When students ask Taoist master Mantak Chia how to deal with their illnesses, he generally tells them: "'Just do the Microcosmic Orbit; this will connect the parts of your body as a whole. Seek balance first, and many problems will be solved.'"[58]

This balance, however, is not static. It is based, rather, on a constantly renewed inner attention to our true physical center of gravity—the lower tan tien, the energy center just below the navel—in the midst of the inner and outer movements of our lives. The rhythmical expansion and contraction of natural breathing, originating deep in the belly, supports this attention and helps activate the energy of this center and circulate it throughout our bodies *for a more complete sensation of ourselves.* As we have seen, it is this overall organic sensation that can help free us from what Lao Tzu calls our "our narrow sense of self," and begin to open us to the alchemical forces of healing and wholeness.

Specialized Breathing Practices

The integration of natural breathing into our everyday lives is perhaps the most practical work we can do on behalf of our health, well-being, and inner growth. We have already explored some of the many physiological effects of such breathing on the various functions of our organism. We have also discussed the salutary effects that natural breathing has on our emotional lives. There is nothing mysterious about the many effects of natural breathing on our lives. They are based on the inner workings of our organisms, on the laws of the Tao, of yin and yang—on the laws of life itself. Through self-observation and self-awareness, we can begin to experience these laws and live and grow in harmony with them.

Once we have begun to practice natural breathing on a regular basis in the ordinary conditions of our everyday lives, there are a variety of specialized breathing practices we can undertake for specific needs. These needs might include cleansing the respiratory system; relaxing in the midst of stress; revitalizing specific organs of the body; getting rid of congestion or headaches; and so on. There are scores of traditional practices to accomplish such goals. In this Appendix, I have included several of my own favorites. Because these practices depend on the ability to sense ourselves and our energies from inside, long practice with natural breathing is generally necessary before we can obtain real benefits from them. An exception to this is the "six healing exhalations," a simple, yet powerful healing practice that can be undertaken by anyone at any time.

157

The "Six Healing Exhalations"

The "six healing exhalations" is an ancient Taoist breathing practice that uses the power of sound to help heal the organs of the body and transform the negative emotions associated with these organs. I first learned this practice from Master Mantak Chia, who calls it the "six healing sounds," and have since come across many references to it in the Taoist canon. Master Chia teaches the six healing sounds in conjunction with specific postures and movements designed to help the sounds reach the appropriate organs. He points out that the "frequencies" of these sounds can help cool and detoxify our organs and speed up the healing process, and maintains that anyone who practices these sounds daily will seldom get sick for very long.[59]

Description of the Sounds

The six sounds are related to the major organ systems of the body, and their associated energy channels. The first sound, "ssssss," the sound of hissing, acts on the lungs and colon, and is related to the nose. The sound is said to be useful for physical problems such as colds, coughs, and congestion and for emotional problems such as grief and sadness. The second sound, "whooo," the sound you make when you blow out a candle, acts on the kidneys and bladder, and is associated with the ears. This sound is said to be useful for increasing your overall vital energy, and for problems such as cold feet, dizziness, and lack of sexual energy, as well as for emotional problems such as fear. The third sound, "shhhh," the sound that you use when you want someone to be quiet, acts on the liver and gall bladder, and is associated with the eyes. This sound is said to be useful for eye problems, anorexia, and vertigo, and for helping to transform the emotions of anger and jealousy. The fourth sound, "haaa," acts on the heart and small intestine, and is associated with the tongue. It is said to be useful for heart disease, insomnia, ulcerations of the tongue, and night sweats, and for transforming emotions such as hatred, arrogance, and impatience. The fifth sound, "whoo" (guttural, in the back of the throat), acts on the spleen and stomach and is associated with the mouth. It is said to be useful for digestive problems, mouth ulcerations, muscle atrophy, and menstrual disorders, and for transforming worry and anxiety. The last sound, "heee" (hissed through the teeth), acts on the triple warmer (the three breathing spaces). It is used to help harmonize the overall energy flow of the body, and is said to be effective for sore throats, abdominal distention, and insomnia.

PRACTICE

To ensure the overall health of all the organs and the harmonious movement of energy throughout the body, the six healing exhalations or sounds should be practiced daily in the order given above. Each sound should each be done at least three times. If you have a particular problem associated with a specific organ or emotion, you can spend more time with the associated sound, repeating it as many times as you like. The practice itself is extremely simple. You can undertake it in any posture. Whichever organ you are working with, sense that you are inhaling energy directly into that organ. As you exhale using the associated sound, simultaneously sense any toxins or excess heat in the organ being carried out of your body with your exhalation. In addition to exhaling audibly, you can also experiment with exhaling inaudibly, concentrating the vibration of the sound inside the organ. The sounds can be practiced safely at any time.

HEAD BREATHING

Head breathing is a little-known technique that can be used to help get rid of headaches or to clear your mind of nervous energy. This practice depends on being able to experience the upper energy centers of the microcosmic orbit—especially the mid-eyebrow point, the crown point, and the jade pillow at the base of the skull—and to sense energy moving through the pathway that connects these centers.

PRACTICE

Sit or stand comfortably. Bring your attention to the mid-eyebrow point. As you breathe in through your nostrils, sense your breath moving your chi from this point up through your forehead and around to the crown point at the top of your head and then down the back of the head to the jade pillow at the base of the skull. As you exhale through your nose, sense your breath moving your chi in the reverse direction— from the base of the skull over the top of the head and back to the mid-eyebrow point (Figure 36). Breathe in this way from three to six times,

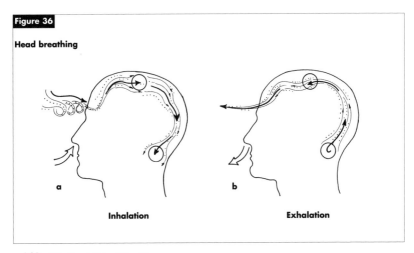

Figure 36

Head breathing

a

b

Inhalation

Exhalation

sensing that each inhalation and exhalation is helping your chi clear the pathway of any stagnation or nervous energy. If you have trouble experiencing your energy moving through this pathway, use your fingers to trace the pathway and to massage these points, and then try again. If you can work in this way without tensing the muscles of your face and head, you will soon experience definite results.

DIGESTIVE BREATHING

Digestive breathing is a simple but effective practice that can help promote digestion. It is based on using your hands to stimulate energy points related to the spleen and stomach meridians, while you simultaneously breathe deep into your belly.

PRACTICE

Sit on a firm chair with your spine erect, yet relaxed, and your feet flat on the floor in front of you. Place your hands on your knees with the heel of your hands above your knee caps and your fingers pointed downward (Figure 37). Use your fingers, especially your index finger, middle finger, and ring

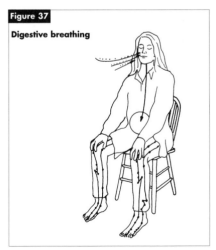

Figure 37

Digestive breathing

finger, to find three indentations in your knee where the fingers can comfortably fit. Your middle finger will be over the center of the knee cap. Now simply keep your hands there, using just a slight pressure to stimulate the meridians running through the knee area. Sense the warmth going into your knees from your hands. As you inhale, sense that you are breathing energy gently into your expanding belly. As you exhale, sense your belly naturally contracting. Do not use force. Work in this way for at least five minutes after each meal, or any time you have digestive problems.

THE TAN TIEN CLEANSING BREATH

The tan tien cleansing breath is a powerful practice for both health preservation and self-healing, as well as for increasing your inner, vital energy. Based on natural, abdominal breathing, it involves directing the breath through the nose and trachea into the lower tan tien, the area just beneath the navel, and exhaling waste products up and out through the nose or mouth while simultaneously condensing the breath energy into the cells of the lower abdomen. The tan tien cleansing breath requires a long, slow exhalation. By intentionally prolonging the exhalation, we not only promote the removal of toxins from the body, but we also help turn on the parasympathetic nervous system, thus furthering deep inner relaxation and healing.

PRACTICE

We have already learned both the theory and practice of abdominal breathing. The key to using tan tien breathing to help heal yourself is to inhale gently all the way down into the tan tien area, an inch or two below your navel. As you inhale, put your attention on the lower tan tien and sense your breath energy filling your lower abdomen. Feel how your abdomen naturally expands. As you exhale, sense any tensions and toxins going out with the breath as your abdomen naturally contracts, but do not, as Mantak Chia warns, "throw out the baby with the bath water." Learn to be attentive to the vital warmth or vibration of the breath energy remaining in your abdomen as you exhale. Guard it with your awareness. Feel it being absorbed deep into your cells as you exhale waste products out through your nose or mouth.

Tan tien breathing is the essence of natural breathing, so be patient and gentle as you undertake this practice. The key is to work with your full attention, without any feeling of willfulness, and to sense the energy in your abdomen. If you can work in this way, the tan tien cleansing breath will quickly become a regular and natural part of your life.

BELLOWS BREATHING

Bellows breathing involves the rapid contraction and relaxation of the abdominal wall to effect exhalation and inhalation, and is a fundamental practice found not only in Taoism, but also in Hinduism, Buddhism, and many other traditions. The practice is designed primarily to help remove various toxins and waste products from the lungs and blood stream. But the practice has many other benefits as well. It helps open and clear the various air passages in the head and throat. It helps pump lymph through the lymphatic system, thus supporting the body's ability to ward off disease. It provides a powerful internal massage of the abdominal area, stimulating the digestive system and oxygenating and energizing all the internal tissues and organs. It strengthens the diaphragm and abdominal muscles, eventually helping them to function more efficiently. And it even helps massage the brain, through respiratory waves transmitted via the circulatory system, specifically through the carotid arteries. And it does all of this without causing us to hyperventilate.[60]

PRACTICE

To prepare for this practice, sit or stand in the basic posture. Put your hands on your belly, and sense your weight sinking downward. Breathe naturally into your abdomen, letting it expand as you inhale and contract as you exhale. Continue in this way until you can really sense your belly from the inside. Now let your chest, and especially your sternum, sink downward. Sense how your chest relaxes as this sinking movement takes place. Take several more abdominal breaths, allowing your chest to remain motionless.

1 Expel the air with sharp exhalations

When you feel ready, expel the air from your lungs through your nose with a strong contraction of your abdominal wall. In other words, exhale by drawing your belly back toward your spine in one rapid movement. The effect of this movement is to push your diaphragm upward, thus expelling air from your lungs. After the exhalation, let your lungs automatically refill themselves without any effort on your part and without any intentional pause. Let the vacuum you have created in your chest do the work. *Your lungs will probably fill to about one-half of their capacity; in any event, do not let them refill completely before your next forced exhalation.* Again, contract your abdominal wall, forcibly expelling the air from your lungs. Put your attention completely on the exhalation; let the inhalation take care of itself. Continue breathing in this way, starting at a rate of one complete breath every three or four seconds and gradually working to a rate of one every second (over many weeks and months).

2 Check for unnecessary tension

The key to this practice is to be sure that your breath is being regulated by your abdominal contractions and expansions. Scan your chest, neck, shoulders, and face to make sure that they remain relaxed. People often grimace when they try this exercise, and the unnecessary tension closes off the nasal passages and constricts the flow of both breath and energy. This can cause headaches and other problems. When you find unnecessary tension any place in your body, smile into it, and start again. Do not continue with bellows breathing if you can sense pain or discomfort, especially in your head, chest, or belly. If you do feel pain, take a break and then start again at the beginning, breathing naturally into your belly with full awareness.

Because bellows breathing involves breathing much faster than normal, many people associate it with hyperventilation. If you carry out bellows breathing correctly, however—using not your chest muscles but rather your abdominal muscles—you will not experience the extreme symptoms often associated with hyperventilation, such as intense dizziness, ringing in the ears, and even fainting. You may, however, especially when you first start bellows breathing, feel some dizziness. This dizziness is not just the result of the change in the oxygen/carbon dioxide balance in your blood, but is also a temporary result of opening the energy channels. If you do feel dizzy, or if you feel you aren't getting enough oxygen, stop bellows breathing, take a long slow inhalation, hold your breath for several seconds, and then exhale. You can do this as many times as necessary. Then start bellows breathing again. At the beginning, start with nine breaths. Then graduate to 18, 36, and so on, over a period of weeks or months until you can breathe for two minutes or more in this way.

Bellows breathing is especially effective in the early morning, in the fresh air, to help jump-start your day. But it can also work wonders when you feel physically, emotionally, or mentally tired, upset, or out of sorts. Whenever you do the exercise, let your belly do the work. Be sure to take clear sensory impressions of yourself both before, during, and after this practice. It is through these impressions that you will improve your practice and understand for yourself the real benefits of bellows breathing.

REVERSE ABDOMINAL BREATHING

Reverse abdominal breathing, traditionally called Taoist breathing, reverses the natural in-and-out movements of the abdomen that one finds in natural breathing. In reverse breathing, the abdomen contracts inward during inhalation and relaxes outward during exhalation. Though reverse breathing offers many of the benefits of natural breathing because of its similar emphasis on moving the abdomen, it is traditionally used by chi kung practitioners, healers, and martial artists to help draw energy deep into their tissues and bones, as well as to direct energy—for storage, for action, or for healing—to any part of their organism. It is also used to build up what is called "guardian chi," a protective shield of energy around the body that helps ward off negative influences, including bacteria and viruses dangerous to our health. It is thus especially useful to help immune system functioning.

Part of the reason for the great power of this practice is the change in the pressure differential between the chest and abdomen. When the diaphragm moves downward and the belly contracts inward during inhalation, the resulting pressure in the abdomen helps "pack" the breath energy into the abdominal tissues and organs, as well as into the spine. When the diaphragm relaxes upward and the belly relaxes outward during exhalation, the sudden release of pressure guides the energy outward wherever one's attention is directed. It is therefore extremely important when undertaking reverse breathing to be clear about where one puts one's attention. Otherwise one's energy may be quickly lost.

In spite of its many benefits, reverse breathing should only be undertaken when one is quite comfortable with natural abdominal breathing. Without this level of comfort, most people who attempt reverse breathing tense their faces, necks, and chests and draw their diaphragms upward as they inhale. This not only negates the positive effects of the practice, but can also lead to a variety of problems, including chest pain, diarrhea, an increase in heartbeat or blood pressure, and energy stagnation. It can also lead to mental and emotional confusion and a scattering of the energy of awareness.

PRACTICE

Though you can practice reverse breathing in a sitting posture, it is best, especially at the beginning, to use a standing posture. This will make it easier to feel your weight sinking and thus will help counteract any tendency to pull your diaphragm upward as you inhale. To prepare for this practice, do tan tien breathing for several minutes, making sure that your shoulders and chest stay relaxed. Also check to make sure that your diaphragm moves downward as you inhale and upward as you exhale. Breathe in this way until you begin to feel a definite warmth or vibration in your belly.

1 Reverse the breathing process

When you feel this warmth, draw your belly slowly back toward your spine as you inhale, and let it relax outward as you exhale. As you inhale, be sure to keep your chest relaxed and to sense your diaphragm moving downward. As it does so, you will feel pressure building up in your lower abdomen, even all the way down to your perineum. If you sense any pressure in your solar plexus area, you need to relax your chest more and to be sure that your diaphragm is moving downward as you inhale. One way to support this relaxation is to let your shoulders move slightly forward and to sense your sternum shifting slightly downward.

2 Guide the energy to specific areas

As reverse breathing begins to become more natural to you, start paying more attention to the quality of the energy being packed into your abdomen as you inhale. As you exhale, allow this energy to expand outward to nourish your entire body. You can also use your attention to help guide this energy to any particular part of your body that you wish to help heal. If you're having a problem in a particular area, continue to inhale into your abdomen, but visualize and sense your breath energy going to the problem area as you exhale.

The Psychological Dimensions of the Microcosmic Orbit

According to Taoist master Mantak Chia, each of the energy centers of the microcosmic orbit influences our emotions in a particular way, depending on the degree to which the center is opened or closed. In my own personal work with the microcosmic orbit, it has become quite clear to me that learning how to sense these various centers, or points, helps open them so that energy can flow more freely throughout the organism. This work with sensation is also a direct path to self-knowledge.

The following outline of the energy centers and their emotional influences (derived mainly from Mantak Chia's teachings and books) is not meant to be exhaustive or final. As you begin to learn how to use your breath to sense your body and emotions in the midst of the daily activities of your life, you may find psychological traits other than those listed associated with these centers. What is certain is that working in this way will bring you to a new understanding of yourself, particularly of the relationship between your physical life and your psychological life.

Navel Center

Taoist sages and Chinese medical practitioners regard the navel center, which includes the lower tan tien, not only as the physical center of the body, but also as the body's main "storage battery" for chi. As Mantak Chia states: "The navel center was our first connection with the outside world. All oxygen, blood, and nutrients flowed into our fetal forms through this abdominal doorway. As a result, the navel center has a special sensitivity that continues far beyond the cutting of the umbilical cord at birth; it stays with us throughout our entire lives."[61]

Closed: One experiences a lack of psychological balance—a sense of being distracted or critical. One is not open to receive new impressions.

Opened: One feels a sensation of openness to the world, a sensation of being centered.

Sexual Center

This center—located for women slightly above the pubic bone and between the ovaries, and for men at the base of the penis about one and one-half inches inside the body—is the basic energy "generator" in the human body.

Closed: One feels an overall lack of energy and little enjoyment from life. One feels self-destructive, negative, and listless.

Opened: One feels a sense of personal, creative power, and the ability to get things done.

Perineum

The perineum is located between the sexual organs and anus. Because of its anatomical position, it connects the two channels of the microcosmic orbit and serves as the foundation for the inner organs of the abdomen.

Closed: One feels insecure and lonely. One also fears any kind of change.

Opened: One feels grounded, rooted to the earth and its healing energies. One also feels a sense of peacefulness.

Sacrum and Coccyx

Though the coccyx and sacrum represent two different locations, we will treat them as one for the purposes of the microcosmic orbit. It is in the sacrum and coccyx that many major nerves from the organs and glands come together, and energy is directed up the spine. It is in this area that the Taoists believe that earth energy and sexual energy are refined and transformed before they move up to the higher centers.

Closed: One feels unbalanced, heavy, and hopeless. One feels that the past is a prison, and that one is under the sway of many unconscious fears.

Opened: One feels light and balanced. One feels that the past is a resource that can be drawn upon for a deeper understanding of and engagement with life.

Kidney Center

The kidney center is located between the second and third lumbar vertebrae of the spine. You can find this point by putting your finger on your spine opposite the navel, and then bending forward at this point. The vertebra that protrudes the most marks the area of the kidney center. Called the door of life, or the mingmen, this center is where our prenatal vitality, our sexual essence, is stored.

Closed: One feels fear and a lack of balance. One also feels a lack of vital energy.

Opened: One experiences feelings of openness, abundance, and generosity.

Adrenal Center

The adrenal center (T11), located between the eleventh and twelfth thoracic vertebrae opposite the solar plexus, lies between the two adrenal glands which sit on top of the kidneys. The adrenal glands, which produce adrenaline and noradrenaline as well as a variety of other hormones, are the primary energy source for the sympathetic nervous system, and are activated whenever there is stress and the instinctive "fight or flight" response.

Closed: One feels either hyper or listless. Old fears can return and begin to shape our experience and behavior.

Opened: One feels a sense of vitality and confidence.

Center Opposite the Heart

This center, which is located between the fifth and sixth thoracic vertebrae between the shoulder blades, has a close relationship with the functioning of the heart and thymus gland.

Closed: One feels a sense of burden and hopelessness. One also feels a sense of chaos.

Opened: One has a feeling of freedom, as well as a deep-felt sense of living.

Center Opposite the Throat

This center, located just below the seventh cervical vertebra (C7), is the central junction box where the energies, nerves, and tendons from the upper and lower parts of the body meet. Any blockage of this center restricts the flow of energy up the spine to the higher centers in the head. You can easily find this point by bending your head forward; the vertebra that protrudes the most is C7.

Closed: One feels disconnected from both oneself and others. One feels a sense of stubbornness and inappropriateness.

Opened: One feels able to embrace both oneself and others with humanity.

Small Brain Center

Sometimes called the jade pillow, this center lies above the first cervical vertebra in the hollow at the base of the skull. This center includes the cerebellum and medulla oblongata, which help control muscle coordination, as well as respiration and heartbeat. For the Taoist, this center is a storage place for the earth force and for refined sexual energy.

Closed: One feels dullness, burden, and suffocation. One may also experience neck pain.

Opened: One feels inspired.

Crown Center

This center is at the top of the head, where an imaginary line from the top of one ear to the top of the other intersects with the midline of the head. This center has a special relationship with the pineal gland, as well as with the thalamus and the hypothalamus. The crown center is connected with the central nervous system, as well as with the sensory/motor system.

Closed: One may fall under the influence of illusions or delusions, losing oneself either in a false sense of pride or the feeling of being a victim. One may have erratic mood swings and headaches.

Opened: One radiates a deep happiness, and feels that one is receiving guidance from higher forces.

Pituitary Center

This center, sometimes called the third eye, lies midway between the eyebrows approximately three inches inside the skull. This center produces hormones that govern a wide range of bodily functions. The Taoists believe that this center is the home of the spirit.

Closed: One feels a lack of aim, of decisiveness. The mind wanders and is unable to make decisions.

Opened: One feels a sense of real purpose, as well as a sense of direct knowing, of intuition.

Throat Center

This center, which includes the thyroid and parathyroid glands, is located in the V-like space at the bottom of the throat just above the sternum. The functions of this center include speech, dreaming, the production of growth hormones, and the regulation of the metabolism.

Closed: One feels choked up and unwilling or unable to communicate or to change.

Opened: One is able to communicate clearly, even eloquently, and one's dreams are more lucid.

Heart Center

From an energetic standpoint, the heart center is between the nipples in men, and approximately one inch up from the bottom of the sternum in women. The opening to the heart center is very small, so this center can be easily blocked or congested. The heart center governs not only the heart but also the thymus gland, which is an important part of our immunological system.

Closed: One feels any one of a variety of negative emotions, including arrogance, self-pity, impatience, and hatred.

Opened: One feels joy, love, patience, honesty, and respect for oneself and others.

Solar Plexus Center

This center is about three-quarters of the way up between the navel and the bottom of the sternum. This center is related to several organs, including the stomach, spleen, pancreas, and liver. It is in the cauldron of the solar plexus that Taoists believe that the sexual energy (ching) and life-force energy (chi) are transformed into spiritual energy (shen). Mantak Chia believes that although it is important for the solar plexus center to be opened, "if it is too open, one may be overly sensitive to the thoughts, feelings, and opinions of others, to the point of being unable to shut off mental and emotional static when in the company of others."[62]

Closed: One feels panic and worry. One is overly cautious.

Opened: One feels a sense of inner freedom, and the ability to take risks on behalf of oneself or others.

NOTES

1 P. D. Ouspensky, *In Search of the Miraculous* (New York: Harcourt, Brace & World, 1949), p. 387.

2 Karlfried Durckheim, *Hara: The Vital Center of Man* (London: George Allen & Unwin, 1970), pp. 154-55.

3 Of course, hyperventilation can be a powerful tool in the work of trans-formation. On pages 170-184 of Stanislov Grof's book *The Adventure of Self-Discovery* (New York: State University of New York Press, 1988), the author, a well-known psychiatrist and founder of "holotropic therapy," points out that sustained hyperventilation helps to loosen psychological defenses and bring about a "profound emotional release and physical relaxation." Grof believes that this occurs not just through the traditional psychiatric mechanism of catharsis, but also because hyperventilation brings to the surface "deep tensions" in the form of "lasting contractions and pro-longed spasms ... that consume enormous amounts of pent-up energy." In Grof's framework, it is the eventual burning up of this energy through these sustained contractions and spasms that brings about psychophysical transformation. This is usually intensely emotional work, and the person undertaking it may require a great deal of individual therapeutic atten-tion. What's more, according to Grof, since hyperventilation initially amplifies and makes manifest the various psychophysical tensions in the organism, it is important to continue this form of breathing until resolu-tion and release take place. As fascinating and important as Grof's work is, it is my intent in this book to show how it is possible to rediscover our natural, authentic breath in the ordinary conditions of life, without the need for psychiatric help. I will not, therefore, explore the therapeutic techniques of hyperventilation any further.

4 See, for example, *The Jade Emperor's Mind Seal Classic: A Taoist Guide to*

Health, Longevity and Immortality, trans. Stuart Alve Olson (St. Paul: Dragon Door Publications, 1992), pp. 69-71.

5   Lao Tzu, *The Complete Works of Lao Tzu,* trans. Ni, Hua-Ching (Santa Monica, Calif.: Seven Star Communications, 1989), p. 14.

6   This "ultradian" rhythm, long observed by medical science, is related to the functioning of the brain hemispheres and can play an important role in healing. When the left nostril is more open, the right hemisphere of the brain is generally more dominant; when the right nostril is more open, the left hemisphere is generally more dominant. One can intentionally open a nostril that is more congested and thus make the other hemisphere more active by lying down on one's side with the congested nostril above and continuing to breathe through the nose. If one is feeling out of sorts or has a headache, trying this experiment for 15 or 20 minutes can often bring relief.

7   Swami Rama, Rudolph Ballentine, and Alan Hymes, *Science of Breath: A Practical Guide* (Honesdale, Pa.: Himalayan Institute, 1979), p. 41.

8   It is interesting to note that some diseases, such as diabetes, can increase the acidity of the blood without increasing carbon dioxide. Since the respiratory center is unable to differentiate the cause of this increase in acidity, it automatically increases the breath rate.

9   Even people with severe pulmonary problems can quickly benefit from work with breathing. In experiments at Shanghai No. 2 Tuberculosis Hospital, 27 people with pulmonary emphysema were able to increase the average range of their diaphragmatic movement from 2.8 centimeters at the beginning of their treatment to 4.9 centimeters after a year of training—an increase in diaphragmatic movement of more than 57 percent. The results are reported in *300 Questions on Qigong Exercises* (Guangzhou, China: Guandong Science and Technology Press, 1994), p. 257.

10   Mantak Chia, private paper.

11 See, for example, Charles Brooks, *Sensory Awareness: The Rediscovery of Experiencing* (New York: Viking Press, 1974).

12 Ilse Middendorf, *The Perceptible Breath: A Breathing Science* (Paderborn, Germany: Junfermann-Verlag, 1990).

13 Rollo May, *Love and Will* (New York: Dell Publishing Company, 1974), p. 237.

14 See, for example, Royce Flippin, "Slow Down, You Breathe Too Fast," *American Health: Fitness of Body and Mind*, Vol. 11, No. 5 (June 1992).

15 For a further explanation of neuropeptides, see Candace Pert, "The Chemical Communicators," in Bill Moyers, *Healing and the Mind* (New York: Doubleday, 1993) pp. 177-94.

16 See, for example, Lawrence Steinman, "Autoimmune Disease," *Scientific American*, September 1993 (Special Issue on "Life, Death, and the Immune System").

17 Ernest Lawrence Rossi, *The Psychobiology of Mind-Body Healing* (New York: Norton, 1988), pp. 173-74.

18 Another effective way to turn on the parasympathetic nervous system is through special movement and awareness practices such as tai chi and chi kung. Among many other benefits, these practices can help release unnecessary tension in the back, especially in the spine, where the main neurons of the central nervous system reside. It is my experience that people with frequent lower back pain are often the same people who have trouble not only relaxing but even admitting that they need to relax. When carried out in the correct way, tai chi and chi kung increase relaxation not only by making the spine more flexible, but also through the deeper breathing that they promote.

19 For further information on the subject of anger, see David Sobel and

Robert Ornstein, "Defusing Anger and Hostility," *Mental Medicine Update: The Mind/Body Newsletter,* Vol. 4, No. 3 (1995).

20 Moshe Feldenkrais, *The Potent Self: A Guide to Spontaneity* (San Francisco: Harper & Row, 1985), p. 95.

21 Peter Nathan, *The Nervous System* (Oxford: Oxford University Press, 1982), p. 48.

22 See James Wyckoff, *Wilhelm Reich: Life Force Explorer* (Greenwich, Conn.: Fawcett Publications, 1973).

23 See Moyers's book, *Healing and the Mind,* particularly the interview with David Eisenberg on the subject of chi (p. 255).

24 Andre van Lysebeth, *Pranayama: The Yoga of Breathing* (London: Unwin Paperbacks, 1983), p. 28.

25 Robert Ornstein and David Sobel, *The Healing Brain: Breakthrough Discoveries About How the Brain Keeps Us Healthy* (New York: Simon and Schuster, 1987), p. 207.

26 For more information on ions, see Fred Soyka with Alan Edmonds, *The Ion Effect: How Air Electricity Rules Your Life and Health* (New York: Bantam Books, 1977).

27 See *The Primordial Breath,* Volume 2, trans. Jane Huang (Torrance, Calif.: Original Books, 1990), p. 13, for a clear description of this very esoteric practice. I will not go into this practice since it is extremely advanced and I have little experience with it. I will, however, discuss in later chapters an associated practice, introduced to me by Mantak Chia, of breathing into and swallowing the saliva.

28 Mantak Chia and Maneewan Chia, *Awaken Healing Light of the Tao* (Huntington, N.Y.: Healing Tao Books, 1993), p. 41.

29 *Awaken Healing Light,* pp. 41 ff.

30 *Awaken Healing Light,* pp. 185-86.

31 Lao Tzu, *Tao Te Ching,* trans. Victor H. Mair (New York: Bantam Books, 1990), p. 69.

32 Taoist reverse breathing often occurs spontaneously for anyone making great physical effort, especially in sports, martial arts, and so on, since it can help to generate outward force through the various limbs. To intentionally activate this form of breathing is quite difficult, however, and can, if done prematurely, cause a great deal of tension and have ill effects on the organism. Before trying reverse breathing it is best to have worked with abdominal breathing for at least several months.

33 Tzu Kuo Shih, *Qi Gong Therapy: The Chinese Art of Healing with Energy* (Barrytown, N.Y.: Station Hill Press, 1994), p. 35.

34 Robert B. Livingston, in *Gentle Bridges: Conversations with the Dalai Lama on the Sciences of the Mind,* eds. Jeremy W. Hayward and Francisco J. Varela (Boston: Shambhala, 1992), p. 174.

35 See pp. 47-54 of *Qi Gong Therapy* for a further discussion of some of the physiological results of respiratory exercises.

36 Chuang Tzu, *Basic Writings,* trans. Burton Watson (New York: Columbia University Press, 1964), p. 74.

37 Alexander Lowen, *The Spirituality of the Body: Bioenergetics for Grace and Harmony* (New York: Macmillan, 1990), pp. 37-38.

38 *Pranayama,* p. 31-32.

39 *The Complete Works of Lao Tzu,* p. 12.

40 *Basic Writings,* p. 138.

41 Tarthang Tulku, *Time, Space, and Knowledge: A New Vision of Reality* (Emeryville, Calif.: Dharma Publishing, 1977), p. 5.

42 *The Perceptible Breath,* p. 32.

43 From an article by Magda Proskauer, "The Therapeutic Value of Certain Breathing Techniques," in Charles Garfield, ed., *Rediscovery of the Body: A Psychosomatic View of Life and Death* (New York: A Laurel Original, 1977), pp. 59-60.

44 Recent biomedical research, such as that reported in Moyers's *Healing and the Mind,* makes it clear that what we think and feel can have an immediate positive or negative impact on our whole body, including our immune system. Of course, Taoism and other traditions have been aware of the influence of our thoughts and feelings on our health for thousands of years.

45 Norman Cousins, *Anatomy of an Illness* (New York: Bantam Books, 1979).

46 Mantak Chia, *Taoist Ways to Transform Stress into Vitality* (Huntington: N.Y.: Healing Tao Books, 1985), p. 33.

47 William James, *Psychology* (Greenwich, Conn.: Fawcett Publications, 1963), p. 335.

48 Moshe Feldenkrais, *The Elusive Obvious* (Cupertino, Calif.: Meta Publications, 1981), p. 61.

49 Paul Ekman and Richard J. Davidson, "Voluntary Smiling Changes Regional Brain Activity," *Psychological Science: A Journal of the American Psychological Society,* Vol. 4, No. 5 (September 1993), p. 345.

50 Phone conversation with Candace Pert, May 9, 1995 (see also note 15).

51 *Taoist Ways to Transform Stress,* p. 33.

52 For a contemporary, detailed description of scientific findings and Taoist beliefs regarding saliva, see the Winter 1993 issue of *The Healing Tao Journal,* Healing Tao Books, P.O. Box 1194, Huntington, NY 11743.

53 *In Search of the Miraculous,* p. 181.

54 *The Healing Brain,* p. 202.

55 From an article entitled "The Body's Guards" in *Living Right* (Winter 1995), p. 23.

56 Master Mantak Chia writes extensively about the microcosmic orbit in his 1993 book *Awaken Healing Light,* and offers readers many practical techniques for opening the governor and functional channels.

57 *Awaken Healing Light,* p. 170.

58 *Awaken Healing Light,* p. 496.

59 See Mantak Chia's book *Taoist Ways to Transform Stress* for the complete six healing sounds practice, including physical movements and postures.

60 My first experience with bellows breathing was highly instructive, since I had not yet understood how to breathe naturally. It took place during a spiritual retreat. On the first day, advanced breathing exercises were given to all of us, even beginners. To be sure, everyone at the retreat was told that these exercises should not be done from the ego or the will, but rather from a state of relaxation and exploration. But being instructed how to do something is not the same as being able to experience it. When we were asked, for example, to do bellows breathing (called *bastrika* in the various Indian traditions), the result for many people, including myself, was almost comical—frantic, spasmodic movements of various muscles all over the body, movements that seemed more willful than

skillful for most of us there. Even many of the more senior students had trouble carrying out the exercise in a harmonious way. As I looked both at myself and those around me, I observed tense faces, necks, shoulders, chests, and arms—psychophysical manifestations of the "upward pull" referred to by Durckheim (see the Introduction)—as many of us tried to do these exercises without the inner relaxation, sensory awareness, and muscle control that are necessary. What was amazing to me was that no one came around to help or correct us. The upward pull became even more evident when the teacher asked us to do bellows breathing, first through one nostril and then through the other. As we continued these pranayama exercises over the course of the retreat, with little visible transformation of these tensions, I began to feel that the teacher had generously overestimated the ability of many of his students to put his teaching into practice. Today, I would simply say that he had not pre-pared his students properly to be able to carry out such exercises in a beneficial way; he had not taken the time necessary to help them learn natural breathing.

61 *Awaken Healing Light,* pp. 173-74.

62 He discusses ways to shield the solar plexus on pp. 245-46 of *Awaken Healing Light.*

INDEX

A

abdomen, energy center in, 81–89, 155, 162–163. *See also* navel
abdominal breathing
normal, 83–84, 90, 93, 162–163
reverse (Taoist), 20, 84, 166–168, 183n. 32
See also natural breathing
abdominal distention, 159
abdominal muscles, 40–42, 100, 164
abundance, 173
acceptance, 50, 51, 115
acid/alkaline balance, 36–37, 180n. 8
acquired chi, 90–91
acupuncture, 78, 148
adenoids, 32
adenosine triphosphate (ATP), 35
adrenal center, of microcosmic orbit, 150, 173
adrenal glands, 58, 173
adrenaline, 58, 62, 173
Advaita Vedanta, 15, 19
aging prematurely, 43
air
components of, 31
movement through respiratory system, 31–33
quality of, 90, 104
alchemy, inner, 81, 99, 149, 155, 176
alcohol, 60
alkaline/acid balance, 36–37, 180n. 8
alternate nostril breathing, 20
alternate nostril congestion, 31–32, 180n. 6
alveoli, 33
amnesia, somatic and emotional, 48
anatomy of breathing, 29–33, 34
anger
autonomic nervous system and, 57

health and, 14
organs and, 132
quality of breathing and, 55
self-sensing and, 57
six healing exhalations and, 158
spacious breathing and, 126
survival value of, 58
venting of, 60–61
anorexia, 158
anxiety
autoimmune diseases and, 57
autonomic nervous system and, 57
hyperventilation and, 54
self-sensing and, 57
six healing exhalations and, 159
spaciousness and, 114
survival value of, 58
aorta, 38
appetite loss, 132
arrogance, 158, 175
arthritis, 56, 57
asthma, 42
ATP (adenosine triphosphate), 35
attachment, 145–146
attention
awakening, 59–60, 66–67, 84–89, 94–95
defined, 85
relaxation response and, 59–60
reverse abdominal breathing and, 167, 168
self-sensing and, 59–60, 66–67, 84–89, 94–95
shen and, 92–95
stress and, 59
See also awareness; self sense
attitudes, 21, 134, 145–146, 147. *See also* self sense
autoimmune diseases, 57
autonomic nervous system, 35, 57–62

awareness
    attitudes and, 21
    clarity and mindfulness and, 20,
    29, 92
    relaxation and, 51, 65
    sensory/organic
    awakening, 69–73
    defined, 47–48
    tension and, 65, 145
    See also attention; self sense; self-
    sensing; spiritual growth

B

babies. *See* infants
back pain, 149, 181n. 18
bacteria, 42, 167
bad habits, 42–43, 49–50, 117
balance
    breathing spaces and,
    116–117, 159
    energy centers and, 83, 155
    healing and, 155
    health and, 64
    microcosmic orbit centers and,
    172, 173
    psychological states and, 145
    See also harmony
balanced breath, 53
baraka, 77. *See also* chi
beauty, rate of breathing and, 35
being, doing vs., 62. *See also* will
bellows breathing, 163–166,
    185–186n. 60
belly
    opening the, 85–86, 89
    outer breath and, 101, 102, 105
birth process, 27–28
bladder, 70, 137, 138, 158
Blake, William, 13
blood
    circulation of, 43, 84, 90
    hemoglobin, 33, 35
    pH of, 36–37, 180n. 8
blood cells, 78
blood pressure, 56, 57, 132
body
    historical, 47

listening to the, 51, 53
    as microcosm of universe, 48–49
    mind and
    chemistry of connection
    between, 55–57
    chi and, 78–80
    parasympathetic nervous system
    and, 59–60
    sensation of, 114–115
    sensing from inside.
    See self-sensing
    somatic amnesia, 48
    wisdom of, 47
    See also organs/tissues
boredom, 53, 55
brain
    breathing into, 94–95
    effort and, 63–64
    energy center in, 81, 92–95
    massaging, 164
    opening the, 94
    rate of activity of, 93
    relaxation and, 64–65, 90, 93
    respiratory center of, 35–36
    self-sensing and, 52, 53
    smiling into, 138–139
    stimulation of
    excessive or inadequate, 60, 146
    need for, 146–147
    tension and, 63
    See also nervous system; neuropep-
    tides; *specific parts of brain*
brainstem, smiling into, 139
breathing
    attitudes and, 21, 22
    bad habits of, 42–43, 49–50, 117
    as buffering mechanism, 15, 29
    chest, 41–42, 54. *See also* shallow
    breathing
    chi and, 77
    deep. *See* deep breathing
    dis-ease and, 17, 42–43
    ecology of, 27
    emotions and, 11, 14, 17, 49, 53,
    55, 134
    energy and, 17, 35, 77
    energy channels reopened by, 148

following the breath, 50–51, 69
harmony and, 17, 42–43, 80
healing and, 17, 18, 20, 62
health and, 11, 14, 15, 17, 18, 27,
  49, 147, 157
holding breath, 20, 27, 36
importance of mastering, 19
inner breath, 35, 100–103, 106
involuntary nature of, 35
mechanics of. *See* mechanics of
  breathing
miracle of, 17
natural. *See* natural breathing
outer breath, 72, 101–103, 105
quality of, 54–55
rate of. *See* rate of breathing
rhythms of. *See* exhalation;
  inhalation
self sense and, 21, 22, 27, 49,
  50–51, 104–105
shallow, 15, 17, 41–42, 54, 100
smiling breath, 129–140
spacious breath, 111–127
spirit and, 77
spiritual growth and, 11, 14, 15,
  18, 49
"taking the breath away," 35
Taoism and, 18, 75–95, 99
three kinds of, 53–54
three spaces of, 115–117, 120–121,
  123, 159
vital breath circulation, 143–155
vitality and, 17
whole-body, 97–109
wholeness and, 17, 27, 62
yin and yang of, 27
yogic complete, 33
yogic techniques of, 19–20
See also breathing exercises
breathing exercises
  abdominal breathing
    normal, 83–84, 90, 93, 162–163
    reverse (Taoist), 20, 84, 166–168,
    183n. 32
  alternate nostril breathing, 20
  bellows breathing, 163–166,
    185–186n. 60
  brain breathing, 94–95

complicated, 20
connecting heaven and earth, 109
counting schemes, 20
digestive breathing, 161–162
following the breath, 69
head breathing, 160–161
hyperventilation, 20, 179n. 3
inner movements of breath, 106
opening body areas, 84–89, 91, 92,
  94, 106, 120–121, 135, 152–154
organ awareness, 71–73
outer movements of breath, 72,
  105
playfulness and, 66, 127
proper approach to, 20–21, 65–66,
  127
releasing deep tensions, 91
retention of breath, 20
reverse breathing
  Taoist abdominal, 20, 84,
  166–168, 183n. 32
  vital breath circulation and, 154
self-sensing, 43, 65–69, 71–73,
  84–89, 105–109
sitting position for, 67–68
six healing exhalations, 157,
  158–159
smiling breath, 135–140
spacious breath, 119–127
specialized, 157–168
spine and
  lengthening the spine, 107–109
  sensing the breath of the spine,
  122–123
standing position for, 66, 67
tan tien cleansing breath, 162–163
tension and, 19, 165, 167
three kinds of breath, 53–54
vital breath circulation, 151–155
warnings about, 19–21, 155,
  183n. 32
whole-body breath, 105–109
will vs. effortless effort and, 62–64
See also deep breathing; mechanics
  of breathing; natural breathing
bronchi, 32, 33, 34
bronchioles, 33
Brooks, Charles, 47

bubbling springs point, 106, 107
Buddha, 27, 132, 145–146, 163
Buddhism, 47, 114, 132
buffering mechanism, breathing as,
15, 29
burdened feeling, 173, 174

C

caffeine, 60
California Pacific Medical Center, 55
calming. See quieting; relaxation
cancer, 56, 78
carbon, 35
carbon dioxide
  alveoli and, 33
  as component of air, 31
  hyperventilation and, 54
  negative ions and, 79
  pH of blood and, 36, 180n. 8
  plant life and, 27
  stress and, 36–37
  as waste product, 27, 35, 36–37
cautions. See warnings
celestial chi, 80–81, 92–95
cerebellum, 138, 139, 174
cerebral cortex, 36
cerebrospinal fluid, sensing,
  122–123, 125
channels, energy, 81, 82, 148–155
chaos, feeling a sense of, 173
chest breathing, 41–42, 54.
  See also shallow breathing
chest cavity, 29–31
chi, 77–91
  acquired, 90–91
  breath and, 77
  celestial, 80–81, 92–95
  energy of, 77, 78–80
  exercises for, 85–89, 91
  guardian, 167
  health and, 78–80, 93–94, 145
  main storage of, 171
  microcosmic orbit and, 149
  movement of, 101–103
  names for, 77
  negative ions and, 79–80
  original, 81–84

saliva and, 136, 138
three treasures and, 80–81
transformation into shen, 81, 176
triple warmer and, 116
wu, 22
Chia, Mantak, 13, 14, 18, 39, 80–82,
  90, 132, 134, 135, 149, 151, 155,
  158, 163, 171, 176
chi kung
  attention and, 85
  breathing practices and, 11, 14
  chi and, 78–79
  microcosmic orbit and, 155
  parasympathetic nervous system
    and, 181n. 18
  practices of, 78–79
  relaxation and, 181n. 18
  reverse abdominal breathing and,
    166–167
  whole-body breath and, 104
children, 11, 17, 29, 84, 99–100
Chi Nei Tsang, 13–15, 100
Chinese medicine, 48, 78, 85,
  116–117, 148, 171
ching, 80–81, 176
Christ, 27
chronic illness, 56, 60
Chuang Tzu, 99, 113–114
circulation
  of blood, 43, 84, 90
  of vital breath, 143–155
clarity, 20, 28–29, 50, 92
clavicles, 41
clavicular phase of breathing, 33
cleansing breath, 53, 162–163
CNT. See Chi Nei Tsang
coccyx, microcosmic orbit and, 152,
  172–173
coercion. See will
cold feet, 158
colds, 56, 57, 158
colon
  location of, 70
  peristalsis of, 42, 90
  sensing the, 71
  six healing exhalations and, 158
  See also constipation; irritable
    bowel syndrome

comfort, 59–60, 85
communication, throat center and, 175
compassion, 55
congestion
  of one nostril, 31–32, 180n. 6
  sinus, 158
conscious embodiment. *See* self-sensing
consciousness, shen and, 92. *See also* awareness; spiritual growth
constipation, 43, 58
cortisol, 56–57
cosmic force, 80–81, 99
coughing, 32–33, 158
Cousins, Norman, 131
criticism, 83, 93, 172. *See also* judgmentalism
crown, making contact with the, 106, 197
crown center, of microcosmic orbit, 150, 152, 174
crystals, 79

D

Darwin, Charles, 132
daydreaming, 83, 93
deep breathing
  cerebral cortex and, 36
  diaphragm and, 38–39, 41–42
  energizing breath, 53–54
  healing and, 62
  phases of breathing and, 33
  positive emotions and, 55
  See also spacious breath
delusions, 174
depression, 43, 56, 117
diabetes, 180n. 8
diaphragm, 38–42
  anatomy of breathing and, 29, 30, 31, 32, 35, 38–39, 101, 102
  bellows breathing and, 164
  compensating for poorly functioning, 41–42
  referral of pain in, 71
  restrictive influences on, 39–41
  sensing the, 72, 86–87

strengthening, 164, 180n. 9
diaphragmatic phase of breathing, 33
diet. *See* food
digestion
  abdominal breathing and, 90
  autonomic nervous system and, 5, 57, 58
  bad breathing habits and, 42–43
  bellows breathing and, 164
  diaphragm and, 39
  emotions and, 57, 58, 59, 132
  helping, 90, 138, 159, 161–162, 164
  sensation of poor, 149
  six healing exhalations and, 159
digestive breathing, 161–162
digestive tract, smiling into, 138
disconnection, feeling of, 174
dis-ease
  breathing and, 17, 42–43
  guarding against, 167
  microcosmic orbit and, 155
  sensing, 50
  space and, 114
  stress and, 56
  vital breath movement and, 148
  See also healing; immune system; *specific diseases*
diseases, chronic, 56, 60
dizziness, 158, 165–166
doing, being vs., 62. *See also* will
door of life, 88–89, 173
dreams, 175
drugs, 60
dullness, 174
Durckheim, Karlfried, 19, 186n. 60

E

ears, six healing exhalations and, 158
earth, heaven and, 103–104, 109
earth force, 80–81, 99, 103, 172, 174
ecology, of breathing, 27
effort, natural breathing and, 20, 62–64
ego. *See* self sense

electromagnetic field, 103–104
elixir fields. *See* tan tiens
embodiment, conscious. *See* body;
 self-sensing
emotional amnesia, 48
emotions
  autonomic nervous system and,
  57–62
  biochemical correlates of, 56
  breath and, 11, 14, 17, 49, 53, 55,
  134
  Chi Nei Tsang and, 14
  defined, 132
  energy and, 14, 61, 145
  eyes and, 135
  facial expressions and, 133
  health and, 14, 60, 61, 145,
  184n. 44
  heart rate and, 57, 58, 59, 132
  hyperventilation and, 54, 179n. 3
  natural breathing and, 11, 14,
  17, 49
  negative
  abdominal muscles and, 40–41
  accepting as "normal", 60
  attention and, 59
  bellows breathing and, 166
  crown center and, 174
  diaphragm and, 39–40
  energy and, 14
  energy centers and, 83
  expansion of awareness and, 51
  expressing, 60–62
  health and, 14, 60
  hyperventilation and, 54
  microcosmic orbit centers and, 151,
  155, 171–176
  natural breathing and, 11, 14
  organs and, 40–41, 132
  physiological effects of, 58
  quality of breathing and, 54, 55
  repressing. See emotions, repressed
  sexual center and, 172
  six healing exhalations and, 158,
  159
  smiling breath and, 134, 139–140
  spaciousness and, 114
  spiritual growth and, 58

  survival value of, 58–59
  Taoism and, 61–62
  tension and, 37, 55, 58
  transforming, 61–62, 132–133
  vitality and, 60, 61–62
  observing, 68
  phases of breathing and, 33
  positive, quality of breathing
  during, 54, 55
  quieting down, 68
  repressed/suppressed, 40–41, 48,
  61, 100
  self-sensing and, 51, 53, 57–62, 73
  smiling and, 132–133
  spaciousness and, 145
  stress and, 57–62
  sympathetic nervous system and,
  57–58, 59
  tension and, 37, 55, 58, 61
  weather and, 49
  See also specific emotions
emphysema, 42, 180n. 9
emptiness, 22, 119
endorphins, 56, 64
energizing breath, 53–54
energy
  attitudes and, 21
  blockages in, 149–151
  body as microcosm of universe
  and, 49
  breathing and, 17, 35, 77
  centers of, 81–95, 155
  channels/meridians of, 81, 82,
  148–155
  cosmic, 80–81, 99
  direct sensation of, 149–155
  earth, 80–81, 99, 103, 172, 174
  effort and, 63
  emotions and, 14, 61, 145
  generator of, 172
  harmonizing overall flow of, 159
  health and, 78–80, 93–94, 145
  heredity and, 81–84
  increasing, 93, 172
  of life itself, sensation of, 115
  microcosmic orbit and, 122–123,
  147–155
  navel center and, 171

orgone, 77–78
perceptual freedom and, 64
self sense and, 115, 146
self-sensing of, 149–155
sensation of, 115
sexual, 80–81, 83, 173, 174, 176
sexual center and, 172
smiling breath and, 139
storing, 166–167, 171
subtle, 77–95
Taoism and, 18, 75–95, 99
tension wastes, 145
universal, 80–81
Western science and, 77
See also chi
enzymes, 64, 78. *See also* pepsin
epiglottis, 34
Esalen Institute, 47
esophagus, 32, 38
exercises. *See* breathing exercises
exhalation
anatomy of, 29, 31, 32, 33, 35–36, 39, 102
balancing with inhalation, 53
distinguishing from inhalation, 100–103
emphasizing inhalation over, 53–54
emphasizing over inhalation, 53
inner and outer breath and, 100–103, 105–106
pause between inhalation and, 123
phases of breathing and, 33
psychological obstacles to full, 118, 119
quality of, 54–55
self-sensing and, 49
significance of, 17, 27, 49
six healing exhalations, 157, 158–159
spaciousness and, 121–122
exhaustion. *See* fatigue
extensor muscles, 37
eyes, 135, 158

F

face, relaxing the, 125, 133, 135–136

fatigue, 43, 51, 53, 117, 166
fear
autoimmune diseases and, 57
autonomic nervous system and, 57
avoidance of feeling, 15
birth process and, 27–28
of change, 172
diaphragm and, 39–40
health and, 14
hyperventilation and, 54
microcosmic orbit centers and, 172, 173
organs and, 132
quality of breathing during, 54, 55
self-sensing and, 57
six healing exhalations and, 158
solar plexus and, 90
See also panic
feelings. *See* emotions
feet
cold, 158
making contact with the, 106
Feldenkrais, Moshe, 63, 132
Feldenkrais method, 19
fight or flight reflex, 41, 54, 57, 124, 135, 173
following the breath, 50–51, 69
food
chi acquired from, 90
immune system and, 146–147
as stimulation, 60
freedom, feeling a sense of, 173, 176
functional channel, 148–149, 153–154

G

gall bladder, 158
generosity, 173
glands, smiling into, 132
golden elixir, 136
gossip, 83
governor channel, 148–149, 152–153
grief, 158
Grof, Stanislov, 179n. 3
groundedness, 172
guardian chi, 167

guilt, 55
Gurdjieff, G. I., 19, 50, 145–146
Gurdjieff Work, 15, 19

H

Hanh, Thich Nhat, 132
happiness, 174
harmonizing overall energy flow, 159
harmony
  attitudes and, 21
  breathing and, 17, 42–43, 80
  effort and, 62–63
  spaciousness and, 114
  See also balance; yin and yang
hatred, 158, 175
head
  making contact with, 106
  opening and clearing passages in, 163
headaches, 43, 149, 160–161, 174, 180n. 6
head breathing, 160–161
healing
  balance and, 155
  breath and, 17, 18, 20, 62
  breathing spaces and, 117, 159
  deep breathing and, 62
  inner awareness and, 13–14
  laughter and, 131
  microcosmic orbit and, 155
  natural breathing and, 62
  self-. See self-healing
  self sense and, 21–22, 155
  shen and, 92, 93–94
  six healing exhalations, 158–159
  smiling and, 131, 133–134
  spaciousness and, 117
  wholeness and, 13–14, 21, 50
Healing Tao, 13, 14–15
health
  balance and, 64
  breathing and, 11, 14, 15, 17, 18, 27, 49, 147, 157
  chi and, 78–80, 93–94, 145
  diaphragm and, 39
  emotions and, 14, 60, 61, 145, 184n. 44

energy and, 78–80, 93–94, 145
energy centers and, 83, 155
microcosmic orbit and, 149
natural breathing and, 11, 15, 49, 147, 157
nature and, 80
negative ions and, 79–80
neuropeptides and, 56, 64, 133–134
self-knowledge and, 56–57
self-sensing and, 47, 48, 56–57, 65
shen and, 93–94
spaciousness and, 114
spiritual growth and, 18
stimulation and, 60, 145–147
stress and, 56–57, 60
tension and, 14
wholeness and, 80
yin and yang and, 64
heart
  diaphragm and, 38, 39
  location of, 70
  natural breathing and, 11
  referral of pain in, 71
  sensing the, 71
  six healing exhalations and, 158
  smiling into, 136, 137
  Taoism and, 49
heart center, of microcosmic orbit, 150, 152, 153, 173–174, 175
heart disease, 56, 158
heart rate
  autonomic nervous system and, 57, 58, 59
  effort and, 62
  emotions and, 57, 58, 59, 132
heaven, earth and, 103–104, 109
heavens, energy of, 80–81, 99, 103
hemoglobin, 33, 35
herbs, 148
heredity, energy and, 81–84
high blood pressure, 56, 132
higher mind. See shen
Hinduism, 163
historical body, 47
holding breath, 20, 27, 36
honesty, 175
hopelessness, 172, 173

hormones, 64, 78, 84
Huang Ti, 18
humanity, feeling a sense of, 174
human potential movement, 47
humor, 131. *See also* smiling breath
Hymes, Alan, 33
hyperactivity, 173
hypertension, 56, 132
hyperventilation
  anxiety and, 54
  bellows breathing and, 165
  as breathing exercise, 20, 179n. 3
  defined, 54
  emotions and, 54, 179n. 3
  stress and poorly functioning
    diaphragm and, 41
hypothalamus, 138, 139, 174

I

identification, 145–146
illness. *See* dis-ease
illusions, 174
immune system, 55–57
  autoimmune diseases, 57
  chi and, 79
  guardian chi and, 167
  heart center and, 175
  reverse abdominal breathing and,
    167
  self-sensing and, 55–57
  smiling breath and, 134
  stimulation nourishes, 146–147
  thoughts and feelings and, 55–56,
    184n. 44
impatience, 55, 126, 158, 175. *See
  also* patience
impressions, need for new, 145–147,
  172
infants, 11, 17, 29, 84
infections, 42, 43
inhalation
  anatomy of, 29, 31, 32, 33, 35–36,
    38–39, 102
  balancing with exhalation, 53
  emphasizing exhalation over, 53
  over exhalation, 53–54
  inner and outer breath and,

100–103, 105–106
  pause between exhalation and,
    123
  phases of breathing and, 33
  psychological obstacles to full,
    118–119
  quality of, 54–55
  self-sensing and, 49
  significance of, 17, 27, 49
  spaciousness and, 121–122, 123
inner alchemy, 81, 99, 149, 155, 176
inner breath, 35, 100–103, 106
inner growth. *See* spiritual growth
inner quieting, 65–69
inner smile, 131–132, 134, 135. *See
  also* smiling breath
insecurity, 172
insomnia. *See* sleep disorders
inspiration, feeling a sense of, 174
integral awareness. *See* self-sensing
intercostal muscles, 29, 30, 31,
  32, 35
intestines. *See* colon; constipation;
  irritable bowel syndrome; small
  intestine
intuition, 92, 175
irritable bowel syndrome, 56

J

jade pillow, microcosmic orbit and,
  152, 174
James, William, 132
jealousy, 158
Jesus Christ, 27
joy, 175
judgmentalism, 83, 90.
  See also criticism

K

kidney center, of microcosmic orbit,
  150, 152, 173
kidneys
  cleansing and energizing, 88–89
  referral of pain in, 71
  sensing the, 71
  six healing exhalations and, 158

effort and, 63–64
new impressions needed by,
146–147, 172
self-sensing and, 52–53, 57–62
See also autonomic nervous system;
parasympathetic nervous system;
sympathetic nervous system
neuropeptides, 56, 64, 133–134
neyatoneyah, 77. *See also* chi
night sweats, 158
nitrogen, 31
norepinephrine (noradrenaline),
58, 173
nose
alternate nostril breathing, 20
alternate nostril congestion,
31–32, 180n. 6
respiratory system and, 31–32, 34,
101
six healing exhalations and, 158
num, 77. *See also* chi

O

opening body areas, 84–89, 91, 92,
94, 106, 120–121, 135, 152–154
openness
kidney center and, 173
navel center and, 172
sensation of, 115
smiling and, 133
See also self sense, expanding the
opposites. *See* yin and yang
organic awareness.
See organs/tissues, awareness of;
self-sensing
organs/tissues
awareness of
awakening, 69–73
defined, 47–48
tension and, 145

bellows breathing and, 164
drawing energy deep into,
166–167
fear and, 132
knowledge of, 19
massage of, 13, 38, 60, 83–84, 164
natural breathing and, 11, 17

negative emotions and, 40–41, 132
reverse abdominal breathing and,
166–167
six healing exhalations detoxify,
158–159
smiling into, 132, 133–134,
136–138, 139
stress and, 40–41, 132
Taoism and, 49
tension in, 40–41
whole-body breathing and, 104
orgone energy, 77–78
original chi, 81–84
Ornstein, Robert, 79, 146
outer breath, 72, 100–103, 105–106
oxygen
alveoli and, 33
bad breathing habits and, 42
as component of air, 31
efficient use of, 37
energy from, 35
hyperventilation and, 54
increasing intake of, 104
negative ions and, 79
pH of blood and, 36
plant life and, 27

P

pain
avoiding feeling, 29, 100
back, 149, 181n. 18
energy blockage and, 149
neck, 174
"no pain, no gain" approach, 48
physical vs. psychic, 14
rate of breathing and, 35
referral of, 69–71
pancreas
location of, 70
referral of pain in, 71
sensing the, 71, 72
smiling into, 137, 138
solar plexus center and, 176
panic, 90, 176
parasympathetic nervous system,
58–60, 90, 162, 181n. 18
parathyroid gland, 175

patience, 175. *See also* impatience
peacefulness, 172
pectoralis minor, 32
pelvis, diaphragm and, 40
pepsin, 42
peptides, 56, 64, 133–134
perceptions, need for new, 145–147, 172
perceptual freedom, relaxation and, 64–65
perceptual reeducation, self-sensing and, 49–50, 53
perineum, microcosmic orbit and, 150, 152, 153, 154, 172
peristalsis, 42, 90
Pert, Candace, 55–56, 133–134
pH, of blood, 36–37, 180n. 8
pharyngeal plexus, 32
pharynx, 32, 34
phases of breathing, 33–34
pineal gland, 139, 150, 174
pituitary center, of microcosmic orbit, 150, 152–153, 175
pituitary gland, 92, 138, 139
playfulness, 66, 127
pleura, 29
pneuma, 77. *See also* chi
polarity, of heaven and earth, 103. *See also* yin and yang
practice, importance of, 19–20
practices. *See* breathing exercises
prana, 77. *See also* chi
pranayama, 19
premature aging, 43
presence, 50. *See also* clarity
pride, 174
primary channels, 148
Proskauer, Magda, 118
psoas muscles, 37
psychic channels, 148–155
psychological obstacles, to authentic breathing, 118–119
psychological problems, hyperventilation and, 54
psychological states
    microcosmic orbit centers and, 151, 155, 171–176
    physical health and, 145–147

Q

qi. *See* chi
Qi Gong. *See* chi kung
quality of breathing, 54–55
quieting
    inner, 65–69
    thoughts, 20, 68, 93
    See also silence; stillness

R

rate of breathing
    of babies, 29
    bad breathing habits and, 42
    effort and, 62
    factors decreasing, 29, 35–36
    factors increasing, 29, 35–36, 41, 42
    pH of blood and, 36, 180n. 8
    resting, 29, 54
    stress and, 29, 35, 41
reality, awareness of, self-healing and, 50, 51. *See also* self-sensing
rebirthing, 28
Reich, Wilhelm, 77–78, 99
relaxation
    abdominal breathing and, 90
    attention and, 59–60
    awareness and, 51, 65
    brain and, 64–65, 90, 93
    chi kung and, 181n. 18
    expansion of awareness and, 51, 65
    eyes and, 135
    face and, 125, 133
    hyperventilation and, 179n. 3
    lower back pain and, 181n. 18
    natural breathing and, 59–60
    parasympathetic nervous system and, 59–60, 90, 162, 181n. 18
    perceptual freedom and, 64–65
    pH of blood and, 36–37
    rate of breathing and, 36
    tai chi and, 181n. 18
    tension and, 64, 116
    vigilant, 64

Westerners and, 19–20
See also breathing exercises;
letting go
repetition, self-sensing vs., 48
repressed emotions, 40–41, 48, 61,
100
respect, 175
respiratory center, 35–36
respiratory illnesses, 43
respiratory muscles, 37–42
diaphragm. *See* diaphragm
extensor muscles, 37
intercostal muscles, 29, 30, 31,
32, 35
psoas muscles, 37
respiratory system, 29–33
rest, rate of breathing and, 29, 36
retention of breath, 20, 27, 36
reverse breathing
Taoist abdominal, 20, 84, 166–168,
183n. 32
vital breath circulation and, 154
rheumatoid arthritis, 57
ribs
anatomy of breathing and, 29, 30,
31, 32, 34, 38, 41–42
opening the rib cage, 72, 87, 89
risk-taking, 176
Rossi, Ernest, 59
ruach, 77. *See also* chi

S

sacrum, microcosmic orbit and, 150,
152, 172–173
sadness, 14, 158
saliva, 136, 138
science, Western, energy and, 77
self-confidence, 173
self-healing
natural breathing and, 20, 49
self-sensing and, 50, 51
smiling breath and, 134
tan tien cleansing breath and, 162
Taoism and, 80
self-image. *See* self sense
self-judgment, 55
self-knowledge, 52–53, 56–57

self-pity, 93, 126, 175
self-respect, 175
self sense
attachment/identification and,
145–146
attitudes and, 21
bad breathing habits and, 49–50,
117
energy and, 115, 146
expanding the
*breathing and, 21, 22, 27, 49,
50–51, 104–105*
*healing and wholeness and, 21–22,
145, 155*
levels of sensation and, 115, 123
lower energy center and, 155
navel center and, 172
need for, 145–147
overview of, 21–22
perceptual reeducation and, 49–50
smiling and, 133
spaciousness and, 115
going beyond the, 115, 123
See also self-sensing
self-sensing, 47–73
as acceptance of what is, 50, 51, 115
actions and senses and, 52
attention and, 59–60, 66–67,
84–89, 94–95
body as microcosm of universe
and, 48–49
defined, 47–48
effects of, 48, 52–53
effortless effort and, 62–64
emotions and, 51, 53, 57–62, 73
of energy, 149–155
energy centers and, 155
exercises for, 43, 65–69, 71–73,
84–89, 105–109
following the breath, 50–51, 69
health and, 47, 48, 56–57, 65
immune system and, 55–57
importance to breathwork, 19, 20,
47, 84–85
inhalation and exhalation and, 49
inner and outer breath and, 72,
100–103, 105–106
levels of, 114–115, 123

trachea, 31, 32, 34, 101
transformation. *See* alchemy; self-transformation
triple warmer, 116–117, 159
trust, 54

U

ulcers, 43, 56, 158, 159
ultradian rhythm, 31–32, 180n. 6
universal force, 80–81, 99, 103
unknown, embracing the, 119
upper breathing space, 116–117, 120–121, 159
upward pull, 19, 186n. 60.
    See also will
uterus, referral of pain in, 71

V

vagus nerve, 35, 38, 59
vena cava, 38
vertigo, 158
victim, feeling of being a, 174
vigilant relaxation, 64
viruses, 42, 167
visualization, neuropeptides and, 56
vital breath, circulating the, 143–155
vitality
    adrenal center and, 173
    artificially induced, 19
    attitudes and, 21
    breathing and, 17
    chi as, 81
    diaphragm and, 39
    kidney center and, 173
    negative emotions and, 60, 61–62
    self-sensing and new impressions and, 147
    sexual essence and, 83, 173
    six healing exhalations and, 158
    spaciousness and, 115
    tan tien cleansing breath and, 162
    See also chi; energy
volume of breath, 31, 38–39

W

warnings, about breathing exercises, 19–21, 155, 183n. 32
weather, emotions and, 49
Weber-Fechner psychophysical law, 63
well-being. *See* health
Westerners
    energy and, 77
    will and relaxation and, 19–20
wheel of life. *See* microcosmic orbit
whole-body breath, 97–109
wholeness
    all-inclusive, 22
    breathing and, 17, 27, 62
    healing and, 13–14, 21, 50
    health and, 80
    perceptual reeducation and, 49–50, 51
    self sense and, 21–22, 145, 155
    going beyond the self sense, 115, 123
    self-sensing and, 50
    spaciousness and, 115
will
    effortless effort vs., 62–64
    negative effects of, 19, 185–186n. 60
    self-sensing vs., 48, 62–64
    Westerners and, 19–20, 28
wisdom of body, 47
wonder, 55, 115
worry, 83, 90, 126, 159, 176
wu chi, 22

XYZ

yang channel. *See* governor channel
yang and yin. *See* yin and yang
yawning, 53
yin channel. *See* functional channel
yin and yang
    breathing and, 27, 157
    defined, 22
    energy of life itself and, 115
    health and, 64